Ungovernable Life

Ungovernable Life

Mandatory Medicine and Statecraft in Iraq

Omar Dewachi

Stanford University Press

Stanford, California

Stanford University Press
Stanford, California

Printed in the United States of America on acid-free, archival-quality paper

Library of Congress Cataloging-in-Publication Data

Names: Al-Dewachi, Omar, author.
Title: Ungovernable life : mandatory medicine and statecraft in Iraq /
Omar Dewachi.
Description: Stanford, California : Stanford University Press, 2017. |
  Includes bibliographical references and index.
Identifiers: LCCN 2016055520 (print) | LCCN 2016056945 (ebook) |
  ISBN 9780804784443 (cloth : alk. paper) | ISBN 9780804784450
  (pbk. : alk. paper) | ISBN 9781503602694 (electronic)
Subjects: LCSH: Medical policy—Iraq—History. | National health
  services—Iraq—History. | Medical care—Iraq—History. | Iraq—Politics
  and government.
Classification: LCC RA395.I72 A53 2017 (print) | LCC RA395.I72 (ebook) |
DDC
  362.109567--dc23
LC record available at https://lccn.loc.gov/2016055520

Typeset by Dovetail Publishing Services in 11/13.5 Adobe Garamond

To my parents,
Ekhlas and Abdulilah

Contents

Preface

The questions that drive this book are inspired by my personal experiences of growing up in Iraq and training as a medical doctor in the aftermath of the 1991 Gulf War. On August 2, 1990, Iraqis woke up to the news of their government's swift invasion and the annexation of Kuwait. Over the following weeks, a coalition of thirty-three countries, led by the United States, had mobilized to "liberate" Kuwait. For ninety days, the coalition pounded Iraq's infrastructure, destroying the foundations of a modern state. Operation Desert Storm targeted government facilities and destroyed electricity grids, telephone lines, the water supply, and sanitation systems. For more than a decade afterward, Iraqis were subjected to one of the harshest experiments of war under UN economic sanctions (1990–2003). The sanctions prohibited oil sales—Iraq's main export—and banned imports of goods, except for limited and selective supplies of medicine and basic food items. Furthermore, Iraq was prevented from importing material to fix its broken infrastructure.

Under the sanctions, Iraqis witnessed an acute deterioration in everyday life as the infrastructure of the state crumbled. Health and development indicators plummeted, and the country's environment was severely scarred. In effect, the sanctions induced an ecology of "state failure," where the besieged state became unable to restore its damaged infrastructure to prewar conditions. This was further complicated by the inability of the country's advanced health-care system to respond to the swelling burdens of the general population's afflictions. The far-reaching and detrimental effects of that war and sanctions—what Iraqis refer to as *al-hisar* (the siege)—were determinative in shaping Iraq's precarious future for decades to come.

In the fall of 1991, I began my studies at the Baghdad Medical College, the country's oldest medical school. I studied and practiced medicine under exceptional conditions and was one of thousands of Iraqi physicians who were witness to the sweeping assault on the physical, social, and political body under sanctions. From my vantage point, the war and the breakdown of state infrastructure were nowhere more obvious than in the collapse of the country's medical establishment and the slipping away of lives in the hospital setting.

In the summer of 1997, I finished medical school and began my residency at al-Madina—Iraq's largest teaching hospital. Like the majority of doctors in the country, I was a government employee charged with the responsibility of providing state-sponsored health care to the country's population. Located in Bab-al-Muadham, al-Madina houses a complex of teaching hospitals and centers, as well as Baghdad's Medical College. With a capacity of about one thousand beds, al-Madina has been Iraq's epicenter for specialized medical care. Upon its inauguration in 1972, international medical experts celebrated the complex as one of the most advanced medical monuments in the Middle East. The large capacity of the complex and its outpatient department made it the main destination for patients from across the country, including referrals from the vast national networks of public hospitals and primary care clinics in Iraq. For decades, al-Madina had been a site for advancements in different fields of medicine and the training of Iraq's reputable doctors—many of whom received their postgraduate training in the West. Al-Madina was in fact the epitome of a decades-long history that had shaped the inception and making of the state since the British Mandate (1920–1932).

When I started my residency at al-Madina, the main general hospital was in a state of remarkable disrepair. This monument of Iraq's medical modernity was unrecognizable due to the lack of maintenance, the cannibalization of its physical structures, and the absence of spare parts for its outdated medical equipment. The hospital's original white and green paint had dimmed to a dark grey. The paneled ceilings leaked from rusting water pipes, bathrooms were dysfunctional, and many hospital beds were broken. Once fitted with top-of-the-line medical gear, such as a built-in oxygen supply and mounted monitors, these became mere decoration. More than half of other hospital equipment had become scrap.

Similar to other government-run places in Iraq during the 1990s, spare parts were scavenged from one machine to salvage another. Patients and their families brought their own bedding to spread over half-torn mattresses, and they were responsible for their own food, and often medicines and medical supplies as well.

My first months of clinical rotation were at the surgical ward. There was a severe shortage of professional medical personnel, and the daily duties of junior doctors, such as myself, compensated for the work of the scarce numbers of the nursing staff. My daily tasks entailed recording patients' vital signs, following up with their medications, and changing dressings when needed. I followed up with lab results and reported the daily conditions of patients to the residents and senior physicians during their morning and evening rounds. For the most part, the main nursing station was abandoned, and only one or two nurses attended to each floor. During night shifts, I would sleep on a broken bed in a room located at the end of the ward, where I was the first to be notified if something happened on the floor during the night, usually by patients' escorts. Such experiences were overwhelming and demoralizing.

Trained in the science and art of modern medicine, textbook therapeutics were becoming obsolete in the face of the lack of medical supplies and the rapid corrosion of the health-care establishment. At the same time, diseases were becoming increasingly unruly. Bacterial wound infections spread with vicious speed and were the primary causes of postoperative deaths. Treating such infections was becoming a menace for the doctors, who had to improvise to deal with the fallout of the limited availability of medications and the mounting septic conditions in this debilitated hospital setting. Many crucial antibiotics were put on the UN sanctions list of banned imports due to their "dual use" for military and civilian purposes. Available options were limited. Regardless of the magnitude of the surgical procedure, it became a common practice to routinely prescribe the only three available antibiotics at government pharmacies to cover the broad spectrum of possible bacterial and fungal infections. Still, the hospital supply of a certain antibiotic would be available one day and not another—disrupting treatment regimens and predisposing the hospital population to further complications. The hospital also lacked regular supplies of intravenous fluids and cannula tubes, urine catheters, sterile gloves, and surgical stitches—essential supplies used in everyday medicine and surgical management. Doctors reused cannulas to economize, replaced urine catheters with nasal tubes to empty bladders, and sterilized disposable gloves and the remains of surgical sutures so they could be used on the next patient. In this mélange of care and toxicity, such improvised practices became essential to saving lives at the hospital ward.

Death was a common sight in al-Madina. Empty coffins went into the hospital's morgue to come out full, accompanied with shrieking screams of mourning. Such screams, unsettling as they were, became familiar. Outside the hospital, clusters of impoverished men and women sat awaiting news about their sick relatives, as they shared their experiences with others. Many of the patients and their families had come from different parts of the country—many were from Iraq's poor provinces and rural peripheries. They had traveled hundreds of kilometers by buses, taxicabs, and private cars to seek essential treatment for their sick family members in the country's largest health-care facility, where the state machinery of maintaining the lifeline of the population had been undermined. Such state failures often manifested in outbursts of violence against doctors led by patients' disenchanted family members.

The breakdown in health care further refracted in the intensifying state control over doctors. Physicians were banned from travel without government approval. At the same time, government bureaucrats and informants monitored physicians closely at the workplace. Hospital administrators would harass doctors in cases of disobedience through bureaucratic and political threats. If caught trying to leave, a doctor would be charged with treason and subjected to six years in prison. Despite the tightening of control, hundreds of Iraq's senior and junior doctors were escaping the country every year. This entailed taking high risks in defiance of the state's travel ban and paying off smugglers to escape the country. Passports were forged and state officers were paid off, as doctors crossing the borders undermined the state's dysfunctional control apparatus. The exodus of Iraq's doctors during the decade of the 1990s, and later after the US occupation of Iraq in 2003, would become a decisive blow to the country's health care.

I escaped Iraq in 1998. I followed the footsteps of hundreds of my colleagues who were leaving the country secretly. I paid off smugglers to renew my passport at the border and left the country unquestioned. Exiting Iraq marked the beginning of a tortuous journey. Many of my colleagues continued their life trajectory to the West. They entered European states both legally and illegally, and applied for asylum as they prepared and sought careers in alternative health-care systems. Unlike them, my trajectory in exile led me to the study of anthropology in the United States—where I lived and experienced the immediate aftermath of the 2003 invasion and occupation of Iraq. Because the 2003 war and occupation became the central event that defined public discourse in the West about Iraq, the impact of the First Gulf War and the sanctions experiment became somewhat obscured. More troubling was the obliteration of a history of a modern nation under ill-informed explanatory models of religion, sectarianism, and authoritarianism.

My aim here and throughout the book is to give readers an insight into Iraq's complex and often obscured history of state building. I have chosen to focus in this preamble on the sanctions as illustrative of a larger theme in this study—that is, of the making and unmaking of Iraq's health-care system. Seeing the sanctions era as a critical event enables us to contextualize the breakdown of this system in relation to a hundred years of medicine and state making in Iraq. Beyond analyzing breakdown and loss within Iraq, this study is a critical intervention in the history and anthropology of medicine, biopower, and governance: an exercise in unraveling the complex histories, topologies, and trajectories of medicine, statecraft, and empire that have shaped life in a region subjected to decades of war, displacement, and destruction.

Omar Dewachi
Beirut, 2016

Acknowledgments

Writing this book has been a project of collective labor and a journey of personal contemplation of the loss of a home. I am grateful to more people than I can possibly list; above all, however, I am indebted to the Iraqis—my family, friends, and teachers—who have taught me the foundations of scientific inquiry and social curiosity, and to all of those who have given me the support, insights, and wisdom needed to complete this ambitious project.

I am grateful to all those who have shared their knowledge and opened doors for me during my fieldwork. Thanks are due to Faleh 'Abdul Jabar, Zeina 'Abdul Noor, Khalid Mohammed 'Abdul Wahab, Dhafer Ahmad, Viqar Ahmed, Yousef 'Akrawi, Tahmima Anam, Azhar al-'Ani, Rana al-'Ani, Shaker al-'Ani, Waleed 'Askar, Ehab Bassem, Ban Bustam, Nicole Le Corgne, Rao Das, Fadhel Derry, Aneez Esmail, Mahmoud al-Hashimi, Ali Jalil, Thura Lutfi, Humam Maki, Ahmad Mousawi, Wisam Mu'een, Omar Najem, Ahmad Naji, Alaa' Nasser, Ahmad Qasim, Ali Rasmi, Ibrahim Rasmi, Omar al-Rawi, Samar al-Rawi, Laith al-Ruba'i, Mohammed al-Samara'i, Hussein Sikaf, Narmeen Taha, Ziad Tariq, Shelagh Weir, Nebras Yahya, Ahmad Zeini, Sami Zubaida, and to Bassel Jabbur, who was my companion in exploring the diverse Iraqi communities in London.

Thanks are in order to Mark Harrison at the Wellcome Unit of History of Medicine at Oxford University for accommodating me institutionally during my fieldwork in the United Kingdom and to the countless staff at the British Library, British National Archive, and the Wellcome Library in London, and the American University of

Beirut, who provided access and assistance to the archives that constitute this book.

At Harvard, many provided me with mentorship, collegiality, friendship, and inspiration. I am grateful to Arthur Kleinman for teaching me to write from the margins and for unending support and guidance; to Mary-Jo DelVecchio Good, Byron Good, Ajantha Subramanian, and Michael Fischer for their invaluable counsel and advice; to Engseng Ho for the stimulating conversations about reimagining history and structure. Mostly, I am thankful to the friendship and mentorship of Steven Caton, who believed in this work and was instrumental in shaping its trajectory.

In Montreal, Canada, I am grateful to the generosity of Margaret Lock, who gave personal and institutional support during the rough patch that came of my inability to return to the United States. I owe much to Vinh-Kim Nguyen, whose mentorship and friendship evolved over the years, and over long walks and cooking feasts. Thanks to Mariella Pandolfi for pushing me to think beyond limits during my postdoctoral fellowship at the Université de Montréal. To those with whom I had long conversations about the project and who have read and commented on its earlier versions: Ryvka Bar Zohar, Caitlin Berrigan, Danielle Carr, Matan Cohen, Michelle Hartman, Louis-Patrick Haraoui, Sam Haselby, Andrew Ivaska, Wilson Jacob, Laurence Kirmayer, Khaled Madani, Chowra Makarimi, Leila Parson, Julie Routhier, Megha Sehdev, Sam Shalabi, and Jonathan Whittall.

Finishing this book would not have been possible without the investment and support of the following institutions: the American University of Beirut, the Ford Foundation, Harvard University, the Wenner Gren Foundation, and the Social Science and Humanities Research Council in Canada.

I am thankful for the support and encouragement of the Faculty of Health Sciences at the American University of Beirut (AUB) and the continuous backing of Deans Huda Zurayk and Iman Nuwayhid. To my colleagues at AUB who have offered their endless support in finishing this book: Ghassan Abu Sittah, Fateh 'Azzam, Monique Cha'aya, Ahmad Dallal, Jocelyn DeJong, Mona Fawaz, Fouad Fouad, Rima Habib, Samer Jabbour, Rami Khoury, Rania Masri, Sylvain Perdigon, Nadya Sbaiti, Kirsten Scheid, Abla Siba'i, Tariq Tell, Jihad Touma, Adam Waterman,

Michelle Woodward, and Livia Wick. My students Mac Skelton, Anthony Rizk, Neil Singh, and Thurayya Zreik have given a fresh perspective on the manuscript. Amir El-Saffar, Omar Isam, Parine Jaddo, Susanne Schmelter, and Hussein Yakoub have offered unconditional support through their friendship and intellectual interest throughout the writing of the book.

Chapters of the book were written while I was a visiting fellow at the Institute for Advanced Study in Princeton during the fall of 2013 and the summer of 2014. Special gratitude is due to Didier Fassin, whose work and insights helped fine-tune the arguments of this book, and to Joan Scott for her interest in the work, critical engagements, and guidance. The argument and chapters of the book benefited from conversations and comments from Hussein Agrama, João Biehl, John Borneman, Ilana Feldman, Elena Glasberg, Sherine Hamdy, Rania Jawad, Joe Masco, Ramah McKay, Lamia Moghnieh, Adriana Petryna, Jasbir Puar, and Noah Salamon.

My journey from medicine to anthropology would not have been possible without the guidance and support of Cynthia Myntti, who introduced me to the discipline and continued to be remarkably generous as our paths continued to cross over three continents and decades. I am thankful to Lisa Hajjar, a true interlocutor and a dear friend who has read my work carefully and provided relentless support. I owe much to Hayder al-Mohammad; our exchanges on theory, life, and Iraq have helped me overcome stagnations and have offered this work sharp intellectual critique and rigor.

My warmest regards go to Kate Wahl at Stanford University Press for her confidence and support from the inception of this book to its completion. I am thankful to the two anonymous reviewers whose critical readings of the manuscript were exceptionally engaging and helped make this a better book. The manuscript has greatly benefited from the close reading, edits, and wit of Jim Quilty.

I am grateful to my partner and muse, Rawya El-Chab, who has been forever generous, loving, and caring in both sickness and health.

My parents, Abdulilah and Ekhlas, to whom I dedicate this book, have supported me throughout my life and career. My father, especially, has been an important inspiration and interlocutor of my work.

Scientists and state-builders like him, who have contributed to the making of Iraq, have become overshadowed by the contemporary discourses that have obscured Iraq's modern history.

Finally, this work is dedicated to all the Iraqis who have suffered and who continue to endure the legacies of war, sanctions, occupation, dictatorship, and exile.

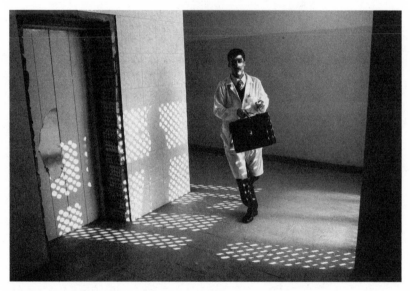

Al-Mansur Children's Hospital in Baghdad, 2002.
Photograph by Thomas Dworzak/Magnum Photos

Ungovernable Life: An Introduction

IN MY DAILY COMMUTE TO WORK, I pass through Hamra Street, the heart of West Beirut's commercial district and nightlife. International shops, such as H&M, Starbucks, and Caribou cafés, line the street alongside smaller local clothing stores, local pubs, and currency exchange booths. The Hamra district is Lebanon's main medical tourism destination and the hub of Beirut's countless private hospitals and medical laboratories. Though the spillover from the armed conflict in neighboring Syria and the fluctuating security situation in Lebanon have deterred many tourists, the neighborhood hotels and furnished apartments still profit from the effects of another regional conflict: an influx of Iraqis in search of health care.

Over the course of my daily wanderings, I have become accustomed to encountering scores of Iraqi patients and their escorts. On one of Hamra's sidewalk benches there is a group of middle-aged Iraqi men chatting about lab results. On the other sidewalk across the street, a woman wearing the traditional Iraqi *abaya* (cloak) is pacing with her sick child. Farther up the street, near Starbucks, a couple of older men dressed in customary robes and *'gal* (headdress) unique to the city of Nasiriyah in the south of Iraq are asking for directions to one of the hospitals. A Lebanese taxi driver, one of dozens parked near small intersections and hotels stalking pedestrians, tells his colleague that he has to go pick up an Iraqi family with a sick family member. Farther down on the main street, two Iraqi men are pushing a wheelchair with a bald child, who is receiving chemotherapy at the local children's cancer center. In Beirut, encounters with Iraqi patients have become troublingly familiar.

In Hamra, the American University of Beirut Medical Center (AUBMC)—one of Lebanon's largest private hospitals—serves a wide range of Iraqi patients. Since the 2003 US invasion and occupation of Iraq, more and more patients from Iraqi cities are frequenting this 400-bed hospital. According to the hospital reports, Iraqis are the second largest national group (after Lebanese) comprising this hospital's patient population. Similar trends are reported from other hospitals across the country. Located near the entrance of the AUBMC is an alleyway leading to the Weekend Hotel—a small seventy-bed inn with a quaint patio. It is just one of scores of small hotels, inns, and furnished apartment buildings dotting Hamra. Since 2007, most of the occupants of the Weekend Hotel have been Iraqi patients and their families frequenting Beirut for a variety of critical medical reasons. In the Weekend Hotel lobby, patients and escorts congregate daily to compare medical updates from the hospital, discuss recent news about events in Iraq, exchange wry remarks about politics, and share personal stories and experiences with others seeking care.

"*Elhayat bil 'Iraq ma'sat* [Life in Iraq is a tragedy]," one chain-smoking escort declares while sipping tea with others in the lobby. He invokes an era of Iraqi prosperity with a blend of pride and defeat. "In the past, Iraqis used to come to Lebanon for tourism," he says. "Now they come for treatment." Next to him sits Abu 'Adel, who had arrived in Beirut to receive his second round of chemotherapy. He explains that he visited a spate of doctors in Iraq before coming to Lebanon. He was first misdiagnosed, then given the wrong medications following incorrect lab results. "In Iraq, there is no state. . . . After years of war, dictatorship, and occupation, we lost trust in our medical system and doctors," he explains, sprawled on the couch after a long and nauseating day at the hospital. "Most of the good doctors have left the country, and those who remain have lost their humanity."

During the 1970s and 1980s, Iraq was celebrated internationally as a "success story"—an oil-rich socialist state achieving universal health care, expanding public health infrastructure, and promoting health among its general population. Doctors received rigorous training in Iraq's internationally respected medical schools, well-equipped hospitals, and research centers. Students from around the region flocked to Iraq to study medicine, and patients from neighboring states traveled there to receive medical care. Today Iraq has become incapable of providing health care to citizens inside its borders, and Iraqis have become disenchanted with the state of their nation's once-vaunted medical system and what many believe is the moral degeneration of the Iraqi doctor.

The phenomenon of patients leaving Iraq in search of health care became widespread after 2003, and took place across Iraq's neighboring countries and their respective health-care systems.[1] In addition to Lebanon, India, Jordan, Iran, and Turkey have also seen increasing numbers of medical care-seekers from Iraq. Moreover, successive post-2003 Iraqi governments have been actively outsourcing treatment of regular citizens, military and security forces personnel, parliamentarians—even members of the country's various militia groups and political parties—to hospitals in Beirut and other regional cities. Still, the majority of patients travel at their own expense in hopes that their journeys will find the life-saving attention unavailable in Iraq. Families sell property and personal belongings, or borrow from relatives, friends, and acquaintances, to facilitate the necessarily frequent visits. Although tens of thousands of Iraqi patients seek medical care outside Iraq yearly, the state has proven incapable of restoring the country's health-care system to the efficiency of its prewar years.

More alarmingly, Iraq's medical enterprise has increasingly been implicated in the political violence and corruption that have plagued the country since the invasion.[2] Since then, attacks on health-care professionals and establishments have become pervasive, and doctors have become the target of far-reaching, organized violence and humiliation.[3] Hundreds of physicians have been murdered or kidnapped by militias and criminal gangs for ransom—some killed in reprisal for their past affiliation with the Ba'th Party, others murdered as a means to further destabilize Iraq's infrastructure.[4] Numerous doctors have been assassinated in their homes or clinics. Others have been targeted with car bombs. In parts of the country, doctors refuse their government assignments or do not show up for their jobs because of insecurity and deterioration of hospital conditions, especially in Baghdad. Across Iraq, doctors have also been subjected to other forms of violence from patients' relatives. Families and kin have taken matters into their own hands, mobilizing party militias or tribal thugs to negotiate with—and if necessary coerce—doctors to pay reparations for a lost life. Fearing retaliation for mishaps incurred during medical or surgical procedures, many doctors have refused to operate on patients.[5] Unable to provide protection for the doctors even inside state-run facilities, the Iraqi government has allowed physicians to carry guns to their workplace.[6] Those doctors who still work in Iraq are at risk and demoralized. Many have urged patients to seek care abroad, knowing that the post-2003 conditions of hospitals pose threats to both patients' lives and their own.

The present state of disarray in Iraq's health-care system does not date from 2003. The systematic dismemberment of the country's medical infrastructure is a product of more than two decades of war and Western interventions, extending back to the US-led Gulf War of 1991 and international sanctions (1990–2003). The sanctions, more particularly, induced an alarming degeneration of the country's health infrastructure and contributed to the exodus of thousands of doctors. Increasing numbers of senior specialists and junior doctors alike have escaped the country, contributing to the further shortage of physicians and expertise. It is estimated that close to half the medical force has escaped Iraq over the past two decades[7]—probably among the largest flights of doctors seen in recent history from one single country. This exodus of doctors is not merely the outcome of war and conflict-induced brain drain. Rather, it speaks to Iraq's complex histories of colonial and postcolonial state building, dating back to the British Mandate (1920–1932).

Ungovernable Life is the first study to document the rise and fall of state medicine in Iraq. The following chapters chronicle close to a century of historical processes, movements, and shifts contributing to the engineering of Iraq's health-care institutions and their eventual dissolution under decades of US-led wars and Western sanctions. The account offers a critique of common assertions about Iraq's state-making histories and of Iraq's dependence on repressive local forms of political rule. It suggests that since the inception of the state under the British Mandate, building the country's medical infrastructures has been a defining feature of a productive mode of governance cultivated and instrumentalized by successive regimes of colonial and postcolonial rule. State medicine in Iraq has never been solely an Iraqi project but one entangled within and shaped by decades of relations with British medical institutions and other international bodies. The making of Iraq's medical infrastructure has been part of transnational networks of knowledge, power relations, and state technologies and practices that politicians and technocrats employed to address a wide range of imperatives and to respond to crises threatening political and social order in the country.

My analysis of this history draws on insights from anthropological and historical approaches to medicine and science as regimes of governance enmeshed in contested colonial and postcolonial state practices and biopolitics.[8] Here, I trace the shifting political role of the figure of the medical doctor across and through the epochs and terrains of Iraq's statecraft.[9] More than any other modern profession in the Iraqi nation-state, the doctor—through the management of national public health—has played a fundamental role in the modernization of the state and the operations of its governing apparatus. Since the inception of the British Mandate, Iraqi doctors have occupied a vital stage in state and nation building. Cultivated as an elite citizen, the doctor has been a vital actor in the normalization of the state in everyday life. Doctors were charged with the delivery of Iraq's universal health care and the administration of urban and rural welfare. Throughout Iraq's modern history, the doctor has also been a critical resource in responding to numerous crises. Medical practitioners have been mobilized to manage endemic and epidemic diseases, to respond to the fallout from development interventions, and to national mobilization at times of war.

Although a product of nation-state imaginaries, the training and professionalization of the Iraqi doctor has been a contested transnational endeavor—subsumed within processes of science and expertise dating back to the British Mandate. Since the inauguration of Iraq's first national medical school in 1927, local doctors have studied under a meticulously designed British medical curriculum and have been supervised by both

Iraqi and British authorities. Over the years, Iraqi and British governments sponsored thousands of Iraqi medical graduates to continue their specialization in the United Kingdom, to build expertise in medical fields, and to expand Iraq's infrastructure. This transaction between Iraq and British health-care infrastructures would continue for decades after Iraq's independence, and it would shape the foundations of institutional life and the career pathways of the country's doctors. During the decades of war, sanctions, and occupation, this enterprise of science and patronage would eventually become one of the catalysts for the dismantling of Iraq's health-care regime. During these years of uncertainty, thousands of physicians fled Iraq and sought security and career opportunities in the British metropole and its National Health Services (NHS), which to date hosts one of the largest populations of Iraqi medical doctors outside Iraq.

By tracing the global histories of Iraq's state medicine and the shifting roles of doctors as agents of state, *Ungovernable Life* offers a fresh insight into the unfolding sociopolitical and infrastructure processes that have shaped the making and unmaking of health care as a form of governance in Iraq. The study delves into the historical processes of medicine and empire that have shaped living conditions during periods of warfare and state dissolution in the Middle East. It attempts to understand how imperial formations of governance, past and present, have intersected, been contested, and parted ways upon the terrain of medicine and state building in Iraq.

Displacing the Gaze

In recent decades, the story of the changing social geographies of health and disease has frequently been told through the lens of states' liberalizing reforms to their health-care systems.[10] It has been argued that the rise of neoliberal doctrine marked the beginning of a "new epoch" in post–Cold War state planning and social welfare practices across the North-South divide.[11] The impact of this doctrine has been increasingly visible, materializing in the deregulation of state governance of the public good in favor of market forces or by moving the locus of governing outside the state.[12] Such deregulation experiments have made states' health-care systems increasingly vulnerable to corporate economies of bioscience, technology, and pharmaceuticals, especially in the global south.[13] Moreover, the rise of humanitarian interventions and the global health enterprise have displaced the state as the sole provider of care, recast citizen bodies and populations in terms of their biological and therapeutic needs,[14] and reframed the management of crisis-struck communities in terms of "bare survival."[15] In response to the undermining of social welfare projects, scholars have suggested that since the onset of this neoliberal "epoch" states' modes of governance and everyday life have become increasingly defined by forms of "abandonment."[16] State retrenchment has become structurally implicated in strategies of rule, in which populations and territories are increasingly governed through ungoverning.[17]

Iraq tells a somewhat different story of state disintegration and ungovernability—one tied more intimately to the histories of colonialism, Western wars, and military interventions in the Middle East.[18] Unfolding in the immediate aftermath of the collapse of the Soviet Union, the 1991 Gulf War and UN-imposed sanctions on Iraq have systematically targeted and destroyed the country's physical infrastructure and undermined its state health-care institutions. While declaring its aim to be the containment of Iraq's war machine after its occupation of Kuwait in 1990, the US-led campaign deliberately targeted civilian as well as military facilities, with the aim of severing the "supply lines" on which the Iraqi regime depended.[19] During the forty-day military campaign, more than ninety tons of bombs were dropped on Iraqi cities, targeting bridges, factories, roads, oil refineries, power stations, and water sanitation and sewage treatment plants. The US military used an array of high-tech weaponry, such as laser-guided bombs, and experimented with depleted uranium (DU) warheads to maximize the destruction of these vital targets. For the next twelve years, Iraq endured what has been described as one of the twentieth century's harshest international sanctions regimes.[20]

The UN sanctions on Iraq were officially designed as a regime of "global governance" and as a containment program aimed at disarming the regime and preventing it from reconstituting its military capacity.[21]

The sanctions prohibited oil sales and banned imports of a wide range of consumer goods, medicines, raw materials, machinery, tools, and the spare parts needed to fix the country's smashed infrastructure. The UN Security Council devised an exhaustive list of items that the Iraqi government was unable to import without UN approval. Items such as chemotherapy medications, batteries, and blackboard chalk were characterized as "dual use"—having a potential use for both civilian and military purposes. The UN Security Council further monitored the flow of goods to and from the country and carried out regular searches of Iraqi ministries and institutions. All states and international companies were obliged to enforce the ban and were prohibited from negotiating deals with Iraq without recourse to the Security Council.[22] States across the global south—in Africa, Latin America, and Asia—structural readjustment programs were increasingly opening state prerogatives to the decentralizing forces of global markets. Iraq's decade-long sanctions regime imposed a different dynamic: it isolated Iraq from the outside world and forced the gradual degradation of the state's social and material infrastructure.

Curbing the Iraqi state's capacity to restore its infrastructure has been described as an "invisible war" with detrimental consequences for the everyday lives of Iraqis.[23] During the 1990s, public health reports pointed out that Iraq, once an effective developmental state, had become a "place of death and sickness." By documenting the scale and scope of infrastructure destruction, such accounts pointed to the everyday suffering of ordinary citizens who bore the brunt of sanctions and the effective dismemberment of decades of state and infrastructure building. According to such accounts, the sanctions regime sent Iraq down a path of "de-development" deteriorating living standards. Reports of rising infant and maternal deaths, widespread food insecurity, and the deterioration of education, health care, and the environment were symptomatic of the "reversals" in development indicators.[24] The sanctions regime, and the concomitant undermining of the state's capacity to govern, further contributed to increasing state violence and brutality.

The US government saw the sanctions as a "failing" to contain the threats of Iraq's authoritarian regime, and the events of September 11, 2011, became a pretext to conclude "unfinished business." The US-led invasion of 2003 was waged under the dubious banner of the

War on Terror in order to eliminate the regime's "concealed" "weapons of mass destruction." In the wake of the fall of the Ba'thist regime, the occupation administration further dismantled state infrastructure by disbanding Iraq's military and police forces. Concurrently—and perhaps consequently—the occupation was marked by the widespread looting of state property, deteriorating security, and eruptions of sectarian violence. Millions of citizens—especially middle-class professionals—were displaced, with close to 5 million Iraqis forced out of the country. Scientists, doctors, and professionals became targets for political assassinations, militia violence, and kidnappings. As the health-care system was overwhelmed by the deluge of those affected by the invasion and its aftermath, outbreaks of disease, epidemics, and fulgurations of violence followed.

Since 2003, media and political pundits have become accustomed to describing Iraq as "ungovernable," using an increasingly familiar litany of tropes to diagnose the spiraling violence and political impasse: authoritarianism, occupation, sectarianism, tribalism, militarization, terrorism, ethnic tensions, et cetera.[25] Iraq's "ungovernability" has been similarly invoked in academic circles, through claims of the inherent fragilities of Iraq—a nation-state supposedly "carved out of the remnants" of the Ottoman Empire after World War I.[26] Iraq, it has been argued, has been made ungovernable by imperial designs that have instilled coercive and spectacular forms of violence as a means of control—a tool, it is claimed, that successive Iraqi regimes used to instill fear and a semblance of order in its population.[27] Alternatively, others have attributed the state of "disorder" in Iraq after 2003 to the nation-state's inability to establish a "foundational myth" and achieve public consensus on its views of the past during decades of state formation.[28] Iraqi society, it has been suggested, has normalized war under decades of conflict and Ba'th Party rule.[29] In such accounts, Iraq seems to have been made ungovernable by strong-willed and violent governments and the "divisions" of a society reawakened by the collapse of the thirty-five-year-old dictatorship of fear that held the country together.[30]

Such simplistic formulations of state making in Iraq could be attributed to ignorance. For decades now, social science research on Iraq has been stifled and fragmented, driven by a dearth of empirical evidence and narrow conceptions of state and society. Scholars working on the Middle East have often overlooked Iraq or studied it from a distance. This has been blamed on restricted access to the country as, since the 1958 revolution, successive regimes have been suspicious of foreign researchers.[31] Others have argued, however, that "scholars of Iraq [in the West] have adopted many practices akin to those used in Cold War Sovietology, relying on a number of instrumental variables that are observable remotely. These include taking the discursive turn in examining the regime's public rhetoric and the historical turn in examining the state's colonial antecedents."[32] Given such systematic inattention and limited, if not flawed, research practices, the study of Iraq has often been "relegated to the margins of social science inquiry,"[33] being "one of the most understudied countries in the world."[34]

Since the 2003 US occupation and the demise of Ba'th Party rule, research on Iraq has faced new limitations. The deterioration of everyday security has made the country a dangerous, if not impossible, site for Western researchers.[35] Furthermore, the large-scale destruction of the country's archives has undermined historical investigation.[36] Like most researchers working on Iraq, I have faced myriad problems associated with limited access to the country and have struggled with the fragmentation and deficiency of available archives.[37] When I started researching Iraq, however, I was perplexed by the dearth of critical analyses of the Iraqi state and the habitual focus on Iraq's Ba'th Party's ideology, violence, and repressive state apparatus. As someone who had grown up, studied, and worked in Iraq as a physician, I found it difficult to reconcile this narrow conceptual framework of the state with the actual complexities of institutional life, and their potential for shaping how the state and the scope of its practices are seen. Although the Ba'th Party's security apparatus was an important instrument of political control, socialization encompassed other forms and processes of state legitimization and modes of governance. My focus on state medicine thus aims to sketch an alternative account of state making in Iraq—one more in tune with the changing relations of state power and its modes of rule. My analysis suggests that, given the country's contested colonial and postcolonial histories, the regimes' shaping of institutional life and population politics has been dynamic, multifaceted, and enmeshed in global processes of knowledge making and power relations. As I demonstrate throughout the book, medical discourses and practices have been central to the country's architectures of governance. Medical schools, state hospitals, government ministries, and overseas educational missions have been sites where state building has been contested and subjects and citizens fashioned.

My criticisms of much of the writing on Iraq that comes from the global north is not only due to disagreement on what the Iraqi State was doing (or not doing). This book argues that new conceptual and methodological tools are needed to analyze state power and its breakdown under decades of US-led wars in the Middle East. Central to this endeavor is tracing and interrogating the different discourses and practices of governance that have imagined Iraq—its geographies, populations, and social institutions—as ungovernable and effectively made it so in swathes of scholarship.

This book demonstrates that discourses of Iraq's ungovernability echo through the different articulations of state making that shaped the country's colonial and postcolonial history. It is my contention that claims of ungovernability are neither mere representational forms aimed to produce an "Other" that is essentially unruly or primitive nor are they responses to modalities of local symbolic orders and alternative medical practices. Ungovernability goes beyond the logic and politics of designation, and is not merely a product of the liberalization of governance. I suggest that ungovernability is tightly enmeshed in the disordered operations of power or, in the words of anthropologist Michael Taussig, "in the tripping up of power in its own disorderliness."[38] In turn, I illustrate how articulations of ungovernability, and the responses to them, became the foundations on which architectures of rule and practices of science and medicine were imagined and deployed in colonial and postcolonial state making. My use of the dialectic of "governable" and "ungovernable" aims to open up new spaces in the analysis of the body politic where we see how regimes of power often produce that which they disavow.[39] Such framing aims to think beyond the dichotomy of power and resistance, as well as recent formulations of governance within economies and zones of exception. My aim is to expand thinking about ungovernability as a feature of the internal dynamics and messiness of power as such.[40] Here, I suggest that the imminent challenge to practices of power and the "will to govern" is predicated on the limits of its internal logics and practices—its own ungovernability. That said, I do not wish to reify ungovernability as a cultural form or a by-product of the particularities of Iraq's state-making history. My treatment of biomedicine and power aims to avoid producing oppositions between modern medicine and cultural practices—as often happens in more traditional accounts in medical anthropology.[41] My framing of power as ungovernable is an attempt to open up and gesture toward some of the internal tensions in the analysis of statecraft, and the refractions of those tensions through different periods of rule and across the dynamics of social institutions. Furthermore, building on the notion of ungovernability, I suggest that one can put together a specific genealogy of metaphors, practices, and careers that links the colony with the metropole and with other colonies—that one might follow people, technologies, and ideas as they move from one site to another. By thinking about the particularities of the Iraqi case and the recent unfolding of conflicts and state collapse in the Middle East, such analysis aims to provide a historically situated counterpoint to recent debates about the changing practices of governance in the so-called neoliberal epoch.

Colonial Disorders

Medical and scientific discourses about the colony as a "place of sickness" and "disorder" are deeply rooted in European and colonial histories and racialized encounters of the nineteenth and twentieth centuries.[42] Emphasizing the role of public health and hygiene projects in colonial governance, historians of medicine have further shown how narratives of colonial pathology were often instrumental in "colonizing bodies,"[43] the molding of colonial subjectivities and race relations,[44] and the control of the everyday conduct of colonizers and colonized.[45] Although the British never officially "colonized" Iraq as they had India, discourses about Iraq as an "unruly place of sickness" trace back to the British military occupation during World War I and subsequent mandatory rule. Prior to the war, the British Empire had questionable intentions in the occupation of Mesopotamia—its term for the Ottoman provinces of

Baghdad, Mosul, and Basra. Mesopotamia had been at the strategic frontier of the Persian and the Ottoman Empires for centuries, but disrupting the politics of the region was an expense no European power was willing to shoulder. During the nineteenth century, British interests in Mesopotamia were mostly confined to the desire to expand maritime trade. On a number of occasions, the East India Company tested the rivers of Mesopotamia as an alternative shorter route linking Europe and the Mediterranean to the Indian Ocean and subcontinent. Such colonial adventures were limited by the fallout from the empire's financial crisis and numerous anticolonial uprisings.

The three-year campaign to occupy Iraq arose from changes in the geopolitical landscape. Soon after the declaration of the war in 1914, and the Ottoman decision to side with Germany, the British Indian government landed a small military force in southern Iraq. The aim of the operation was originally to protect British interests in the Persian Gulf and prevent the Germans from seizing control of oil resources and water navigation around the region. London was reluctant, but the India government saw many benefits to advancing northward to secure the territories. As the occupying force advanced on Baghdad, it suffered a series of military setbacks and medical scandals. Attempts to reach Baghdad from the south failed abjectly after the Ottoman army laid siege to the British Indian force in the southern town of Kut al-'Amara. British efforts to break the five-month siege failed, and disease and mutiny among the Indian soldiers contributed to the force's surrender. In fact, more soldiers died from sickness than actual combat. Responding to what became known as the "Mesopotamian scandal," the British opened political investigations and mobilized mobile hospitals and medical staff to the Mesopotamian frontier and strengthened supply lines to evacuate the wounded.

British accounts of the Mesopotamian campaign often invoked the harsh environmental conditions facing the military. British medical discourse depicted Mesopotamia as an ecology hostile to military occupation.[46] Reports described Mesopotamia's "notorious unhealthy climate, subject to the ravage of practically every known form of infectious disease in an endemic and epidemic form."[47] Military doctors analyzed Mesopotamian ailments from the framework of "tropical medicine."[48] British troops were put under strict medical and hygiene regulations.[49]

Still, commanders and personnel suffered a range of medical and psychological complaints, including heat stroke and exhaustion, cholera, malaria, as well as a range of inexplicable ailments that were seen as related to the country's environmental and geographical conditions. For British officers on the ground, the success of any political project in Mesopotamia had to first reckon with health ailments and mobilize resources to control the threats posed by the local ecology. Colonial and medical officers in Mesopotamia reminded their superiors that the survival of any project depended on the expansion of health care and sanitation to the general population. The Indian government resisted any expansion of the civil administration, but Mesopotamia's military authorities insisted on recruiting more British doctors and health-care staff to establish a comprehensive medical and public health administration that addressed the health of the local population. With mounting anti-British sentiments across the country, building Iraq's new civilian health infrastructure was to be a means for absorbing popular resentment—one contrasting with British attempts to quell local uprisings through use of force.

One of the main concerns of British rule in Iraq after the war was management of medical crises as a function of sustainable state building. After the declaration of the British Mandate in 1920, tropes of Iraq's hostile ecology gave way to the logic and practices concerned with expediting processes of state building and cultivating economic activity. With a relatively small civil administration, the tasks of the mandatory power in Iraq included the creation of a national government and institutions run by local elites under British supervision. Another task was ensuring the economic survival of the new state by integrating Iraq into the imperial economy. As a result, the British invested heavily in modernizing transportation infrastructure to facilitate the flow of goods and people in and out of the country. They opened new roads, laid down railway tracks, and expanded river navigation to cultivate the empire's postwar economic recovery. On a discursive level, the tropes of tropical medicine gave way to the state-building narratives that then preoccupied medical establishments in Europe. British doctors in Iraq emphasized state welfare logics and the centralization of health-care infrastructure, and they called on the Iraqi government to focus on disease prevention and cutting down on economic waste.

Although such discourses represented a shift from conventional colonial medical narratives, they continued to be implicated in the broader processes of the empire's postwar economic recovery. The earlier attempts to create an Iraqi Ministry of Health failed due to the lack of finances and British unwillingness to hand over public health matters to local doctors. Instead, a team of British and Iraqi physicians ran a modest Directorate of Health under the auspices of the Iraqi Ministry of the Interior that was, more or less, under British control. The directorate's work focused on laying the foundations of the new state's health policies and rationale. From the start, the directorate was charged with expanding Iraq's health services and infrastructure, collecting and producing vital statistics, and reporting developments in the country's health care to the British Civil Administration. It monitored the transportation systems closely and created a specialized unit to oversee health and medical matters pertaining to the expanding Iraqi Railways network. The work of the directorate was often challenged by lack of resources and required a more comprehensive system to contain the emerging threats of fast-moving epidemics. British doctors often argued with government elites for the need to centralize the country's underdeveloped and fragmented medical structures. Due to the lack of central government finances, Iraqi officials argued for relegating the running and maintenance of peripheral health care to the provincial authorities.

The British saw centralizing Iraq's health-care administration as necessary to the vitality of the new state and for governance under the rapid modernization of national infrastructure. Paradoxically, the enhanced mobility that resulted from the rapid upgrade of the country's transportation network also made it possible for disease to spread more quickly. British concerns about the threats disease posed to Iraq's fledgling state were exemplified during the cholera epidemic of 1923, which coincided with the annual Shi'a pilgrimage to the holy sites of Karbala and Najaf. During the epidemic, British and Iraqi authorities confronted the shortcomings of simple quarantine procedures and the want of local resources to manage disease. The mobility of the pilgrims—thus the income of the holy cities—became dependent on the new transport infrastructure. Banning the pilgrimage that year would have had numerous political and economic repercussions, especially given the unrest in the south of Iraq following the 1920 anti-British revolt, which had been sanctioned by religious and tribal authorities. Managing the epidemic challenged the new state's capacity to reconcile its economic and security priorities with those of public health. Unable to prevent the movement of pilgrims across the country, the directorate experimented with vaccines flown from India and drew on other imperial resources to carry out a door-to-door vaccination of the Karbala's inhabitants and pilgrims both from inside and outside the country. Directorate activities and the mass production of the vaccine in the newly established central laboratory were further centralized in Baghdad. The successful and swift management of the epidemic was taken as a lesson in the importance of centralizing health-care administration in the capital. It refuted earlier arguments among Iraqi political authorities about the need to decentralize the country's regional hospitals and dispensaries, both administratively and financially. The epidemic also reminded the authorities of the need to cultivate national resources to respond to imminent medical threats to the political, social, and economic orders.

Discourses and debates about Mesopotamia's "unruly" environment underscored the fragilities of the colonial political order. They highlighted the limits of imperial structures in maintaining the health of British and Indian bodies under compromised British military control and in mobilizing medical resources to sustain the mandatory state in Iraq. As I aim to show throughout the book, such discourses of ungovernability often refracted through the practices of postcolonial statecraft. Moreover, the production of contested "pathologies" and "disorders" were often entangled with the political, economic, and technological interventions concerned with the engineering of the state, its environments, and its populations as a polity and a mode of social life.

Mandatory Medicine

Britain's cultivation of Iraq's medical infrastructure was originally a product of anxieties pertaining to neutralizing the military fallout of the Mesopotamian occupation. The British Mandate wanted to create a self-governing state—staffed and operated by Iraqis and supervised by British experts. In fact, the League of Nations Mandate was designed as a regime of "tutelage" that aimed to transform and reorient Iraqis, and their social institutions, toward "rational" processes of state and citizenship making. Central to the mandate's state-building logic was the reconfiguration of broader networks and terrains of science and patronage—where the training of the Iraqi medical doctors would be shaped by long-term connections with British medical institutions after independence.

Historians of medicine have shown us that the introduction of health-care regimes in colonial settings have often engendered projects of different scales and given life to dynamic relations of power that shaped science and governance practices in postcolonial settings, as well as in the metropole.[50] Using the term *postcolonial* as a signpost, Warwick Anderson reminds us that "[a] postcolonial approach means we recognize how modern science and biomedicine are put together, assembled, on the terrain that various sorts of colonialism have worked over—whether in Asia, Africa or Europe."[51] Building on such insights, my analysis will trace how medical infrastructure was assembled on Iraqi terrain. Thus, I use the terms *state medicine* and *mandatory medicine* interchangeably: first, to refer to the distinctive and formative relationship of science and state-making logics and practices cultivated during the mandate; second, to gesture to the ways medicine was bound to the professionalization of medical doctors as state functionaries; third, to emphasize the expanding role of medicine as a regime of biopolitics and governance within the broader social life in the country. To historicize the evolution of mandatory medicine is not to fall into the production of a national history, or a historiography, of science. My analysis of mandatory medicine is more concerned with illustrating how competing global and local powers continued to shape Iraq's state and medical infrastructure-building projects during the post-mandate era. I further show how the interplay of knowledge, technologies, and expertise between Iraq and Britain continuously blurred the lines between center and periphery in the casting and recasting of medical discourses and practices of Iraq's ungovernability.

Central to the analysis of mandatory medicine and statecraft in Iraq is an understanding of the transnational infrastructures of training and professionalization of the Iraqi doctor. It is important to recognize that the British did not "invent" Western medicine in Iraq. The Ottoman Empire had long developed modern institutions and training for local medical doctors across the region during the nineteenth century. That said, under Ottoman rule, none of the provinces of Iraq had a medical school. The handful of locals trained in medicine at the time of the inauguration of the state had received their training in regional medical schools in Istanbul and Beirut. As Chapter Three shows, the "local" doctor in the Ottoman context was less a territorialized national figure than a mobile agent trained in one province and working in another. Ottoman doctors usually traveled where their careers took them and worked in different administrative and military enterprises of the region's different competing empires. Thus, the efforts during the mandate to create a national institution of science and medicine to train Iraqi doctors highlighted the British efforts to realign the networks of science and medical authority to conform with their own. As a result, the training of local doctors under the mandate became predicated on the cultivation of doctors, not only as experts of knowledge and techno-politics,[52] but also as a mode of sociality and citizenship that is produced and regulated by regimes of power and tutelage both in Iraq and Britain.

The inauguration of the Royal College of Medicine in Baghdad in 1927 became a turning point in the development of Iraq's nation-state, being one of the first institutions devoted to professional education in the sciences. The Royal College became the first to train local Iraqis in Western medicine under British supervision.[53] Upon its inauguration, the school was staffed with mostly British doctors, in hopes that, in time, an all-Iraqi faculty would replace the British one. The training of the doctors at the Royal College entailed the creation of a professional world where locals would develop reverence for Western science and train to become citizens and civil servants of the Iraqi state. Students from different parts of Iraq went to train at this state-sponsored medical school. They received free medical training in return for the promise of years of government service in public hospitals and clinics across the country. The language of instruction was English, and the school followed British curricula and education standards. The college cultivated doctors to become cosmopolitan, specialist, and Western oriented through training both inside and outside Iraq. To help inculcate diverse expertise in science and medical disciplines, both the Iraqi and British governments offered their graduates scholarships to pursue their training in the United Kingdom. In turn, doctors were expected to return to Iraq to take over from their British mentors and expand the human medical resources of the state in medical education and in the various specialties of biomedicine needed to develop the Iraqi medical system. Up until the end of the 1950s, British doctors continued to supervise the training of Iraqi medical students and set the standards for medical education and practice in the country. Even when political relations with Britain were strained after the fall of the British-backed monarchy in 1958, Iraqi doctors' association with the imperial metropole remained as strong as ever. The training of Iraqi medical graduates in the United Kingdom was crucial to the production of the elite Iraqi doctor, whose scientific link to metropolitan institutions gave him or her a great deal of leverage over those who remained in the country. Such institutional links further shaped Iraq's transnational practices of science and education, which became governed under the patronage of British medical institutions during the independence period. It further defined the career mobility of doctors between Iraq and the West.

Under the nation-building logic of mandatory medicine, doctors were charged with bringing Iraq into step with modern nation-states through medical science and public health policy. The training of the Iraqi doctor entailed a dual rationale: that of producing the modern citizen and that of improving the governance of the nation's health. On the one hand, advancing expertise in medicine, science, and the production of Iraqi medical professionals was meant to bring the state up to speed with other modern nation-states. On the other hand, doctors carried the responsibility of bringing the countryside into the realm of the state through obligatory provincial government service. In the decades that followed the establishment of the Royal College, state medicine confronted the tensions inherent to its postcolonial state-building role. The government expected young graduating doctors to live and work in underserved areas with the aim of extending the reach of the state to the rural peripheries where state control was weak and endemic diseases prevalent. Although the government expected physicians to go "backward" to provide care for rural areas and focus on the peasantry's ailments, it was in the service of a larger project of "progress" and modernization. Even as they were caught in the tense logic of backwardness and modern progress, doctors were often reluctant to serve in rural areas despite political pressure from—and contractual obligations to—the state. The obligation of medical school graduates to serve in Iraq's rural regions meant Iraqi governments would always run the risk of losing the doctors to other health-care systems. The Hashemite state's inability to develop comprehensive rural health-care infrastructure would have serious repercussions on the state-building project—especially during the Iraqi oil boom of the 1950s and the adoption of nationwide urban and rural development practices.

Revolutionizing Medicine

The health-care infrastructure of Iraq underwent further elaboration following the overthrow of the Hashemite monarchy. At different junctures in Iraq's postcolonial history, other transnational forces were instrumental in expanding and transforming the scope and reach of state public health and social policies. Two critical periods that I explore in this book are the transition from the British-backed monarchy to the socialist era (1958–1980) and the Iran–Iraq war of the 1980s. As I show in Chapters Five and Six, the fallout from these episodes in Iraq's social history—what anthropologist Veena Das might call "critical events"[54]—played a definitive role in the further integration of the "therapeutic" role of the state in the management of broader social and economic aspects of its population. Medicine became one of the central platforms of social and economic reform after the 1958 revolution and an instrument of nationwide mobilization during the brutal eight-year conflict with Iran. This account aims to show how therapeutic discourses of ungovernability and questions of sickness and pathology transcended their biomedical usage and came to be employed in social and economic policies and interventions.

Like many nations in the global south, Iraq's mid-twentieth-century embrace of international development logic and interventions has been a contested undertaking with social, political, and technological facets. From the monarchy through the Ba'thists regime, succeeding Iraqi governments embraced developmental reforms as political and technological strategies to modernize the state and transform society and the economy. Such transformations have been further shaped by the Cold War geopolitics and entangled with the social dynamics and contestations of state building. Iraq's embrace of international development logic is traced to the immediate aftermath of World War II (1939–1945). At the time, the monarchy's state-building practices were overwhelmed by Western and Iraqi elites' fears of swelling antigovernment sentiment and the rising influence of Bolshevik ideologies among the population, including the urban middle classes and rural peasantry. In response to political demands to address rising social and economic inequality, Western and Iraqi experts proposed technical fixes, centering on modernizing the country's urban and rural infrastructure. These included the expansion and development of the country's urban centers to accommodate the rising middle classes, as well as the implementation of large-scale irrigation projects in order to utilize Iraq's undeveloped rural and agricultural peripheries, where most of the country's population resided. The introduction of irrigation projects was conceived as a technological solution to the temperamental behavior of the Tigris and Euphrates rivers whose flooding represented a serious threat to urban structures and harvests.

Soon after the inauguration of irrigation projects, public health experts warned of the potential fallout from non–medically supervised development. The new damns, irrigation canals, and river reservoirs were contributing to the spread of waterborne ailments among the peasantry and compelling mass rural migration to the cities. Public health experts criticized the unsupervised development plans and warned of the medical risks associated with the migration of "peasant pathologies" into the urban centers. Efforts to tinker with the country's rural ecology were further complicated by the peasants' extremely harsh working and living conditions under the local feudal system, better known as 'iqta'.

Development programs were further compromised by naive conceptions of the complex socio-economic processes that defined the

country's rural-urban divide and how these were affected by modernization imperatives. Prior to the 1950s, peasant transhumance from rural to
urban settings had been part of regular patterns of seasonal labor migration. Peasants often moved to larger centers to seek menial jobs during the
agricultural off-season or during extreme conditions such as drought or
flooding. By the mid-1950s, hundreds of thousands of rural migrants had
permanently moved to Baghdad, living in informal settlements erected
on government wasteland along the Tigris River. Uprooted by miscalculated technocratic practice and seduced by the increasing economic
opportunities in the capital, migrants sought temporary and permanent
work in the city's expanding urban infrastructure and government institutions. The inability to contain rural-urban migration raised many red
flags among state officials and development experts, and it provoked
discussions about the incompatibility between urban and rural life. In
contrast to "docile" city dwellers, Iraqi migrants were seen as plagued
with "backward" tribal values that made them defiant of state authority.
Such conceptions echoed through debates about the cultural tensions of
state building and turbulent engineering of Iraqi citizenship.[55] International and local accounts of Baghdad's informal settlements described
the abject physical, social, and environmental conditions of the migrants
and their dwellings. Paradoxically, the implementation of nationwide
development initiatives contributed to the further decline of agriculture
in the country and fueled public resentment against the monarchy. The
fallout from the 1950s' development initiatives became political capital
for succeeding regimes.

The centrality of expanding medical infrastructure into the
countryside became more visible in the public policies of the Qasim
regime. The July 1958 revolution, led by army officer 'Abdul Karim
Qasim, ended thirty-eight years of British-backed rule in Iraq. The
revolution is considered a turning point in Iraq's modern history and
state-making practices. The short-lived republican era (1958–1963)
witnessed major social and economic transformations. One of the challenges facing the revolution was to reverse the fallout of a decade of Hashemite national development policy. In an attempt to improve the social
and economic conditions of Iraqi agriculture, the Qasim government

immediately issued decrees abolishing the feudal *'iqta'* system and reforming land tenure. At the same time, the revolutionary government commenced rapid expansion of state infrastructure and welfare. It introduced a national plan to build a large neighborhood project in the capital and offer public housing to homeless migrants and the poor. The project, which became known as al-Thawra City (Revolution City), materialized before the completion of its service infrastructure and well beyond its intended capacity. In time, al-Thawra City turned into Baghdad's largest urban ghetto. While contributing to stratified urban class formations in the capital, the project further resulted in the depletion of agricultural modes of life. More farmers abandoned their land and headed to the city with hopes of integrating into state welfare and finding better economic opportunities.

Despite setbacks, medicine and medical infrastructure were expanded into the management of wider aspects of social life. Succeeding Iraqi governments inaugurated new medical schools, public hospitals, and dispensaries. It made medical education more available to students coming from the different Iraqi provinces and instituted a quota of students from the different Iraqi governorates. It also introduced new laws to enforce and regulate rural service by medical school graduates. Promising to maintain the traditions of Iraqi medicine, the government continued to offer scholarships for study in the United Kingdom and created new connections with the Soviet Union and other East Bloc states to foster expertise in socialized medicine and public health. Under republican rule, the government carried out Iraq's first national smallpox vaccination campaign with the help of Soviet medical teams. In addition to vaccinating children and adults across the country, the teams trained Iraqi staff in conducting door-to-door surveys and inoculations.

The expansion of medical infrastructure and the instrumentalization of medicine in governance continued under the Ba'th regime, with medicine becoming a central plank in the Iraqi state's social and economic platform. In the 1970s, the Ba'th government nationalized the oil industry, making more funding available for development initiatives and the expansion of state welfare programs. During the decade, the government further expanded medical training programs, and the number of medical doctors in the country grew. It also initiated national literacy campaigns—especially in the countryside. By the end of the decade, the state had effectively enforced elementary education among the country's children and claimed almost 100 percent literacy rate. During the 1980–1988 conflict with Iran, maintaining the achievements of the 1970s—particularly as concerns public health—became central to state policy.

The Iran–Iraq war ended the country's short period of oil-fueled economic prosperity. Soon the country's oil funds were depleted, and the prolongation of the war challenged Ba'thist development policies. The human and economic cost of the war prompted alternative social policies focused on mobilizing the country's human resources for continuing state development practices during the conflict. With medical expertise reoriented to the theatre of war, the government looked for alternative resources, namely the country's women, to ensure the survival of the nation and state infrastructure at wartime. State policies encouraged childbearing and the protection of infants and children in the face of massive human casualties in battle. These policy strategies had a lasting impact in redefining the role of women in society and contributed to their broader incorporation within the labor force.

With the help of UN public health expertise in primary health care, the state harnessed the country's main women's organization—the Federation of Iraqi Women, the feminist arm of the Ba'th Party—to institute a nationwide campaign targeting child mortality. Its aim was to extend vaccination programs across the country and promote low-cost interventions to prevent diarrhea—the main cause of infant and child mortality in the country. The state offered training programs to the country's midwives, enlisting them to report mortality and morbidity in urban and rural areas.

The campaign's success was hailed internationally as an exemplary story of wartime development. Despite the widespread economic and human cost of the conflict, by the end of the war Iraq had reduced the rate of infant and maternal mortality by half and expanded primary care services to different parts of its rural periphery.[56] Furthermore, the war contributed to the cultivation of Iraqi doctors with a wide range of medical and surgical expertise.

The war also consolidated the reach of an authoritarian state that often negotiated both repressive and productive forms of power in shaping Iraq's state-making project. This developmental "victory" would be seriously challenged by the Gulf War and international sanctions of the 1990s, when the widespread destruction and systematic dismantling of the country's health-care infrastructure contributed to a sharp increase in infant and maternal deaths.

Doctors as Infrastructure

The engineering of what I call "mandatory medicine" in Iraq should be read as the story of statecraft and infrastructure development.[57] Over decades of modern state building in Iraq, medicine played an instrumental role in the transnational circulation of people, knowledge, and technologies, as well as connecting centers of power—not only within the postcolonial state, but between center and peripheries of the empire. Since 1991, this infrastructural nature of state medicine has been highlighted in the undermining and dismemberment of the country's infrastructure by war, sanctions, and occupation. The flight of medical professionals who have been integral to the country's architecture of rule has been one of the central tragedies of Iraq's health-care system, signifying not merely the loss of critical state resources but of a mode of sociality that had been cultivated over decades.

The mass exodus of Iraqi doctors over these past decades should be understood in relationship to the legacies of war and state dissolution. During this time, Iraq's doctors had been at the forefront of a war targeting both the state infrastructure and the social fabric of the nation. Medical professionals struggled to address the direct and indirect effects of this assault. They faced economic sanctions, the US invasion and its aftermath, the violence of the state, and the collapse of the health system. As the Iraqi state was dismantled and the alliance between the state and the doctor dissolved, physicians had to negotiate both their presence in and absence from Iraq, as well as the reconfiguration of modes of sociality that extended beyond the borders of the state. As I show in the final chapter of this book, the story of Iraqi doctors did not end with crossing the national border. Despite the travel ban on doctors in Iraq and the international restrictions on travel facing Iraqi citizens, many doctors undertook asylum journeys to Europe, where they sought work, training, and citizenship.

This flight of doctors from Iraq was shaped by the broader quest for training and job opportunities abroad. Leaving a "broken" health-care infrastructure, they sought to find refuge in a "functioning" system that offered the potential of universal medical knowledge, up-to-date technology, and the opportunity to find fulfillment in their chosen field. The path to asylum in the United Kingdom was often dangerous, involving costly payment to human traffickers. In the United Kingdom, Iraqi doctors sought to relinquish their Iraqi papers and to settle. They were lured by the promise of a better life and a career, in what many recognized as the extension of the professional world they knew from their medical training in Iraq.

The story of state medicine in Iraq comes full circle in the United Kingdom. Once trained by Britain as agents of state building, Iraqi doctors found themselves implicated in an overlapping story of colonial disorders—no longer at the periphery of the empire but at its heart. In the United Kingdom, Iraqi doctors came to realize the confines of the empire and its promises. Once agents of science and patronage networks that bound Iraqi medicine to the metropole, their relationship to Britain now had to be reconfigured to the hierarchies and inequalities of Britain's postcolonial health-care system while struggling with asylum claims and fulfilling licensing requirements. Financially constrained, doctors hoping to compete for limited training positions in the UK health-care system sometimes spent years preparing for professional and language qualification exams. Iraqi doctors confronted the reality of an "ailing" Western welfare regime that has been dependent on and partial to "foreign" doctors—especially those from the former colonies.

As this book was being written, there were close to 5,000 Iraqi doctors living and working in Britain's National Health Services (NHS). Thousands more were dispersed in health-care systems across the world. Iraqi doctors' flight to Britain is not merely a story of "brain drain" or "brain gain"—as it is depicted by conventional public health accounts. The movement of doctors to the erstwhile imperial metropole is a consequence of a turbulent century of imperial and post-imperial state making. Founded during Britain's imperial moment in the region, Iraq's medical community and health-care infrastructure were harnessed to a state-building project that was subsequently undone by later waves of international intervention in the region. The Iraqi doctor seeking employment in London, an Iraqi health-care infrastructure smashed by war and sanctions, the Iraqi patient seeking care in Beirut—this is how empire looks in our present-day reality.

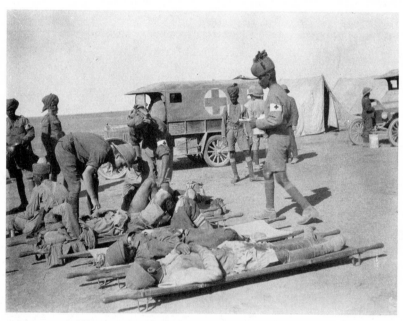

A Royal Army Medical Corps officer tends to a group of wounded Turks on stretchers with the assistance of some Indian staff at an advanced dressing station after the action of Tikrit, 1917.

Photograph by Ariel Varges. © Imperial War Museums (Q 24440)

1

Intervention Pathologies

Isaiah writing of Mesopotamia, speaks of the "glory of king-
doms, the beauty of the Chaldees' Excellency." A recent report
describes the same region as "a miserable wilderness of barren
desert, alternating with vast swamps." Such is the change that
has been wrought in the course of time.

"Mesopotamia," a handbook prepared under
the direction of the historical section of the
foreign office for the delegates attending the
post–World War I Peace Conference, 1920[1]

THE OTTOMAN STATE had just entered World War I on the side
of Germany. It was November 1914 when the British landed an Indian-
soldiered division—the Mesopotamian Expeditionary Force (MEF)[2] near
Basra on the Persian Gulf. Within two weeks, the MEF was in control
of the whole city. The campaign was initially intended to be a holding
operation to protect the imperial interests around the head of the Persian
Gulf. A German-Ottoman alliance threatened Britain's trade and communications with India and endangered the oil fields in Abadan, under
control of the Anglo-Persian Oil Company. Furthermore, the new Ottoman Oil Company in Mosul promised that recently discovered fields in
the north would fall into German hands. Five months later, the occupation turned into an ambitious campaign to occupy the three provinces of
Ottoman Mesopotamia.[3]

After initial reluctance in London, the British government of India
sent General John Nixon to Mesopotamia to order the new division's
commander, General Charles Townshend, to advance north toward
Baghdad.[4] This relatively small division of around 11,000 men, mostly
Punjabi Muslims, faced minimal resistance from the Ottoman army

until it reached al-Mada'in, about 26 kilometers southeast of Baghdad. Al-Mada'in delineated the southern borders of the city of Baghdad as marked by the ruins of the imperial Ctesiphon. It is said that this was once the largest city in the world—one of the Mesopotamian capitals of the Parthian (247 BC–224 AD) and Sassanid (224–642 AD) empires of ancient Persia. During its glory days, it connected trade routes between the Persian Gulf and the Silk Road. It was an object of several short-lived Roman conquests during the first and second centuries.

In November 1915, the ruins of Ctesiphon were witness to one of the definitive battles of World War I. The German general Baron von der Goltz led the 18,000-strong Ottoman force that engaged the British Indian division in a ferocious battle. After three days, his forces exhausted their enemy and caused major casualties. Close to 4,600 men were killed from the British side—almost 40 percent of Townshend's force. Faced with imminent defeat, Townshend ordered the southward retreat of his remaining forces. The general decided to enter Kut al-'Amara—a small town of 6,500 inhabitants located on the Tigris River about 160 kilometers south of Baghdad. He aimed to hold positions there awaiting supplies and reinforcements from Basra.

For 147 days, the Ottoman army laid siege to the river-encircled town, cutting off the force from food and reinforcements. The Tigris was in its flood season, and several attempts to break out across the river on floating bridges failed. Desperately, the British Royal Flying Corps attempted airdrops of food and munitions to the besieged army. The Ottomans shot down the low-flying aid planes before they reached their target. The British command in Basra ordered river transport from London to relieve the expedition. None showed up due to the breakdown of communication and delays related to the ongoing military reorganization at the War Office in Bombay. Heavy rains and the muddy terrain further undermined efforts to free Townshend and his troops. The siege of Kut became a huge setback for the British leadership. It attempted to negotiate the British division's surrender and offered a compensation of nearly 2 million pounds if the Ottomans lifted the siege. Such offers were rejected.

Townshend faced further problems from the locals. Fearing future retaliation from the Ottoman army, Kut's inhabitants refused British commanders' demands to feed the exhausted and famished troops. Local shop owners refused to accept paper money in exchange for the much-needed food. Townshend began to force the locals into submission with flogging and on-the-spot executions, setting an example for others. To further demoralize the besieged army, the Ottoman command snuck Urdu- and Hindi-language pamphlets into Kut, urging the mostly Muslim battalion to abandon their posts, kill their British officers, and join their Muslim Ottoman "brothers."[5] At least seventy-two Indian soldiers deserted, and scores more died trying. Those who were caught attempting to kill British officers had their trigger fingers amputated.

Despite these brutal attempts to gain control, the British Indian unit surrendered on April 29, 1916. During the siege, the battalion lost approximately fifteen men daily to dysentery and another twenty to starvation and heat exhaustion. Many more died in Ottoman captivity after the surrender of the town to the Ottoman army. Close to half of the 8,000 prisoners died on the 1,125-kilometer march from Kut to the Ottoman prisons in Aleppo. By the end of the standoff, the British had lost thousands, mostly to starvation, dysentery, heat exhaustion, and other sicknesses that plagued the campaign. Describing one of the horror scenes of the evacuation of the sick and injured during the operations, one medical officer wrote:

> Out of the haze there emerged a dirty little river paddle steamer, which moored alongside and discharged onto the hospital ship a load of the most wretched humanity possible, all Indian troops, wasted to skeletons by disease, a grim foretaste of what might be expected in a land whose hostility to man was well known, even to the ancients. The river steamer, without any preliminary cleaning up, then proceeded to absorb onto her filthy decks the personnel of an entire hospital unit, and steamed away untidily into the haze.[6]

British discourse of Iraq's unruliness is deeply rooted in the mobilization of military medicine during World War I. The campaign represented one of the war's most controversial military endeavors. One British historian described the defeat of Kut al-'Amara as "the most abject capitulation in Britain's military history."[7] Military authorities blamed this capitulation on the breakdown of medical provisions and communication in preparation for the advance to Baghdad—what became known in Britain as the "Mesopotamian scandal."[8] The scandal prompted serious investigations into the medical and health organization of the British military, and the War Office in India was accused of neglect. As others have shown, experiences of sickness and death in Mesopotamia had a critical influence on instigating broader medical reforms across the empire's war fronts.[9] In Mesopotamia, it also revived an old imperial desire to subjugate the place that went beyond the war's immediate geopolitical interests.

Reigning over Mesopotamia

In a paper read before the Hunterian Society at St George's Hospital, London, in February 1920, Dr. Bailey stood in front of an eager crowd waiting to hear about his experience as a medical officer during the Mesopotamian campaign. News of the scandal had tainted the opinion of many of the medical professionals who were curious about a firsthand experience of the campaign. Supported with images and maps, Bailey first explained the context of the occupation of Mesopotamia in 1914, before sharing his experience of Mesopotamia itself. He told the audience: "There is probably some truth in the saying that all one ever wishes to see of Mesopotamia can be seen through the port-hole of the Steamer."[10]

World War I was not the British Empire's first unruly encounter with the land and its ecology. Mesopotamian territories had been on the radar of imperial interests for at least a century before the war. During the early 1800s, the East India Company proposed to explore river navigation in Mesopotamia as an alternative route to maritime trade between India and Europe. Another strategic goal was the expansion of waterway patrolling to protect the company's vessels from the increasing numbers of pirate attacks around the Persian Gulf. Still, the relatively shallow and tortuous courses of both the Tigris and Euphrates rivers represented a critical technical challenge for ship navigation. The company's newly developed interest came on the heels of the invention and popularization of steamboats during the late eighteenth and early nineteenth centuries. The newly built iron steamers ran on coal and were capable of speedy travel upriver, which had been considered impractical for older wooden ships.[11] The steamboats promised to revolutionize river travel and trade by opening new waterways and shortening travel time between metropole and entrepot.

In 1830, Artillery captain Francis Rawdon Chesney set off on the first expedition to navigate the Euphrates on newly constructed river steamers.[12] After convincing the British government of the urgency of exploring this alternative route, he embarked with two steamers—appropriately called the Tigris and the Euphrates—both built by the East India Company and transported in pieces over land from the Mediterranean to the Euphrates. The expedition's aim was to experiment with rebuilding the two steamers and sailing them downstream to the Persian Gulf. The experiment was a partial success. One steamer (the Tigris) hit underwater shoals and sank. The other never made it to the Persian Gulf, though it remained in Ottoman waters.

Almost ten years later, the East India Company renewed its interest in charting and patrolling of the Tigris. The British had already strengthened their presence in Ottoman Mesopotamia through the integration of mail service with India. The British also constructed telegraph lines from Baghdad to Bombay, Constantinople, and Tehran.[13] The company appointed Henry Lynch to succeed Chesney as the commander of the remaining steamer, the Euphrates. In 1840, Lynch and his brother founded the Euphrates and Tigris Steam Navigation Company, better known as the Lynch Company. Based in Baghdad, the Lynch Company functioned as the trading branch of the East India Company.[14] Soon the Lynch Company secured Ottoman permission for its expeditions and began operating a number of steamers that ran between Baghdad and the Persian Gulf. Despite the failure to establish alternative trade routes through the two rivers, one of the main goals of controlling the waterways was strategic—to protect nearby British establishments from the rising Russian interests in the region.

Lynch was entrusted with the task of systematically surveying the topologies of the two rivers and producing maps for navigation. For the next few decades, he attempted to survey both rivers and prepared charts to explore the possibilities of defining a river route from Basra to the northern city of Mosul. Lynch developed detailed maps of the lower parts of the Tigris, many of which were published in the *Journal of the Royal Geographic Society of London*.[15] These maps' importance went beyond the scientific and commercial spirits of the project. As part of the arrangement with the Ottoman government, it was agreed that the maps would be used only for commercial and trading purposes. Still the Royal Geographic Society frequently updated British military intelligence about these surveys.[16] Lynch often referred to this predicament in his writings. In his account of the 1839 survey of the Tigris River from Ctesiphon in al-Mada'in to Mosul, he wrote, "There could be no difficulty in marching armies along these rivers in the present day; and I must confess I find more difficulty, the more I see of these countries, in reconciling the account of the Greek and Roman campaigns with the actual state of them."[17]

Decades later, Lynch's maps became instrumental in the Mesopotamian campaign. In 1916, the political scandal led to the transfer of command from Delhi to London. This represented one of the main game changers, "one result of which was a massive influx of resources."[18] On December 1917, General Stanley Maude took charge of the Mesopotamian campaign and authorized the advance of 50,000 men from Basra toward Baghdad. The British also mobilized hundreds of hospital ships and thousands of river steamers to provide medical support to the advancing army, running the supply lines back and forth up the river. Empty steamers were used to evacuate the sick and wounded, swiftly clearing military lines for the advance of troops to Baghdad. Many of these steamers were hurriedly constructed in British shipyards or mobilized from different parts of the empire. Describing the scale of this mobilization, one medical officer wrote:

> [A] host of small vessels of every description were dispatched under their own steam from all parts, from Irrawady and Ganges, stern-wheelers from the Nile, and even little paddle steamers from Tyne and Thames, and in the van of this fleet were those same little boats that used to ply the waters of London with holiday crowds. Close to eighty of those steamers were lost en route, overwhelmed by the high seas or sunk by hostile gunfire.[19]

Reigning over the rivers of Mesopotamia had long been an imperial dream and a challenge to the empire's resources. This dream was realized during the war. The occupation of Mesopotamia celebrated the steamer as the embodiment of British improvisation and the empire's technological superiority in securing the medical front.[20] Doctors, nurses, mobile hospitals, and ambulances were mobilized from different sites to expand the campaign's medical infrastructure and to respond to troop demoralization. Within months, the number of hospital beds increased dramatically. In the seven months leading to Maude's advance, the need for hospital beds on the Mesopotamian front increased from 4,700 in January to 15,745 in July 1916.

Despite the major improvements in postwar Mesopotamia's medical organization and sanitation, the British were just beginning to reckon with the country's everyday medical realities. The imminent breakdown of the imperial regime was articulated in anxieties about the psychological and manpower expense of colonizing the place.

Disenchanted Tropics

Late one afternoon in January 1918, the *Minnetonka*—a hospital ship sailing from Malta bearing medical supplies to the Mesopotamian front—dropped anchor at the Bar of Fao on the Persian Gulf. Because the ship was too large to pass north toward Shatt al-Arab, the confluence of the Tigris and the Euphrates Rivers, it awaited transshipment. Two smaller river steamers from the British India Steam Navigation Company carried the 65 British General Hospital (BGH), a 500-bed tented hospital previously located in Malta, along with its staff from Fao to Basra. The 65 BGH was being moved to equip a newly constructed military hospital on the bank of the Tigris. The steamers arrived in Basra, and the staff was transported to a camp in the outskirts of the city. They spent three weeks in transit camps before the orders came, and then they restarted their journey to Baghdad.

The river journey took three days. For most of the hospital staff on board, this was their first tour of service in Mesopotamia. Among those on board was Major Harry Sinderson, a young Scottish doctor serving in the Special Reserve; his first glimpse of land had been "through field glasses from the bridge of the *Minnetonka*" prior to their arrival:

> Mesopotamia was "terra incognita" to everyone on board the Minnetonka. Our pooled knowledge of its geography, people and religion was meager, and Army Headquarters in Greece were unable to add much to it. Such information as was available was not minimal, but far from complimentary. "Mespot" had acquired an unenviable reputation for heatstroke, dysentery, Baghdad Boil and bilharsiasis, among a host of other disorders, infections and infestations common to tropical and subtropical climes. And, too, there had been a *scandilum magnatum* in the previous year, in which charges of inadequate medical and kindred supplies had been levied against army chiefs in India. . . . We all knew, of course, that Mesopotamia was steeped in Old Testament, Assyrian and Babylonian history; that within it was the traditional site of the Garden of Eden; that it was the scene of the familiar exploits of Jonah and Noah, that Ur on the Euphrates was also the birthplace of Abraham and that Nebuchadnezzar's Hanging Gardens of Babylon had been one of the wonders of the world. We were also aware that Alexander the Great had died there and that Baghdad, its capital, well over a thousand years earlier, had been the home of the Abbasid Caliph, Haroun-al-Rashid, his popular fame evinced by the "Arabian Nights."[21]

During the occupation, many of the Mesopotamian "ailments" were seen through the lens of the "tropics." The use of *tropical* in a nontropical context was not uncommon in such colonial military campaigns. Different colonial powers have often mobilized "tropical medicine" as a regime of governance in different settings. As has been argued, the "metaphor of tropical indicated a general dependency on a harsh natural determinism among a population trapped by climatic and geographical conditions."[22] Sinderson's account of his "first encounters with Mesopotamia" is telling of the conflicting historical imageries available for military and medical men during the campaign. "Mespot" was the land of the biblical myth, an enigma to empires that have risen and fallen on its land. Such thickness of history stood in contrast to its present state of decay. Mesopotamia stood for the cradle and grave of civilizations.

Baily's accounts about his own steamer journey were colored with such suggestions. In one account, he describes his visit to what was claimed to be the site of the Garden of Eden—in a small town of Gurna on the confluence of the Tigris and the Euphrates. His steamer had been on its route from Basra to Baghdad in 1917. Baily describes the place to his colleagues at the Hunterian Society in London with some irony:

> The village consists of about three hundred mud dwellings, with a line of more pretentious buildings on the riverfront. Legend has it that Kurna [Gurna] is the site of the Garden of Eden. A white doorway, shaped like a pear, set in a wall of yellow brick, marks the supposed site of Paradise, whilst a bare Tree with small, apple like fruit, growing behind the wall, is said to be descended from the Tree of Knowledge of Good and Evil. . . . Kurna has a reputation of possessing the hottest and most humid atmosphere in Mesopotamia, and produces a severe form of Malignant Malaria. . . . I am of the opinion that if there is anything in the legend about Eden, that there was ample excuse both for Adam and Eve in such a place. At the same time there is no accounting for tastes and Eden may have deteriorated, but the British inhabitants, at any rate, do not require the services of an angel with a flaming sword to drive them from the spot.[23]

In his turn, Sinderson also further elaborates on the daily "disillusions" between the myth and reality:

> I had grown up picturing the "City of the Caliphs" as truly a "dim, moonlit, city of delight." I was bitterly disappointed and painfully disillusioned. Not a vestige of magnificence or affluence; mean buildings; shabbiness that affronted me; and the women who passed by, veiled figures in black, did nothing to illuminate the scene. The concealment of features was a source of annoyance to our soldiery. They assumed it to be due to ugliness and coined for them the expression, "hooded horrors."[24]

Although deeply "racializing" discourses shaped their depictions, Baily and Sinderson's accounts suggest the deeper confusion that characterized the state of "disorder" in which many found themselves. This confusion further metabolized in the semi-scientific and medical explanations of everyday conditions in the country. The country's climate and the landscape in particular were seen to threaten the body and vitality of British and Indian soldiers alike.

Counter-Attractions

The war was coming to a close in Mesopotamia. The expansion of the British occupation and the need to maintain order in the military were imperative for British medical officers. Many were still unclear about the long-term commitments in this place. Both British and Indian servicemen were eager to return home to their families and prewar jobs. Sanitation practices were rigidly enforced among the troops. Commanders tried to insulate the troops within isolated enclaves to minimize contact with the general population. With fears of endemic diseases such as the bubonic plague, movement in and out of the compounds was strictly regulated and regimes of hygiene were installed inside them. With fears of syphilis and other sexually transmitted diseases, the British extended some of their quarantine provisions to entertainment in Baghdad and other major cities under their control.[25] Despite such measures, afflictions like heat stroke, malaria, and other parasitic infections such as skin leishmaniasis were unavoidable.[26] These could incapacitate the soldiers and further threaten fragile troop morale. Such fears were translated into invocations of the environmental risks contributing to servicemen's physical and mental breakdown. Medical officers were trying to rationalize these frequent events.

Prior to the mid-nineteenth century, theories of contagion usually used in tropical medical discourses depended heavily on ecological readings of disease causality. The miasma theory, for example, held that diseases were caused by noxious "bad air" that emanated from decaying organic matter in the surrounding environment—such as foul air, contaminated water, and poor hygienic conditions. The emergence of the germ theory in the mid-nineteenth century never fully uprooted the theory of disease etiology from geography in tropical medicine. As others have clearly shown, "[d]espite the tendency in the new tropical medicine of the late nineteenth century to eschew climate and topography in favour of bacilli and protozoa, there remained a sense in which the physical and the social peculiarities of Africa, Asia and the central regions of the Americas, continued to inform the medical discourse and praxis."[27] In Mesopotamia, too, British doctors were confronting radical transitions in the theory of disease causality from environmental determinism to germ theory.[28] Doctors on the ground confronted an array of conditions that they believed were environmentally produced. Such environmental determinism reflected the experiences of the military campaign and the uncertainties about the future of the colonial project in Iraq. Sinderson's ambivalence about the tropical explanations captured just that. Commenting on the contradictions of the climate and its relationship to the state of health in the country, Sinderson wrote:

> The climate of Iraq combines a number of remarkable contrasts, and one of the meteorological characteristics of its middle and southern regions is the very high atmospheric temperature which persists throughout the summer. The temperature of a country's air remains a major factor in the prevalence of those of its endemic diseases and ailments which are widespread in hot climates and are commonly labelled tropical. Such an expression from a geographical point of view is of course limited to territories between the tropics of Cancer and Capricorn. Geographically, Iraq is a continental subtropical territory, but the fervid heat of its summers exceeds that of most tropical regions. However, the majority of diseases which prevailed in Iraq, but not in temperate climates, are common throughout the tropics, and the label tropical is at least a convenient if not a very accurate description of them.[29]

For Sinderson, both microbial and environmental interactions made up the incongruous ecology of disease in Mesopotamia, where heat was paradoxically both the "poison" and the "cure." He wrote:

> With few exceptions, the diseases of temperate climates are to be found also in tropical and other lands exposed to torrid aestivation, and so it was that in Iraq one met with diseases familiar to the medical profession at home as well as ailments of particular prevalence in glowing climes. As in temperate zones, most diseases are due to a specific cause, commonly microbic, and it is the effect of temperature in such cases that determines to a great extent the diversification of endemic diseases of temperate and tropical climates. . . . Direct exposure to the sunlight adds

to the effect of intense heat and Iraq is indebted to the great luminary for its invaluable contribution to preventive medicine within her borders. Without her scorching solar rays the incidence of infective diseases would surely soar.[30]

Despite such rationalization of the complexities of disease causality, everyday realities of the occupation more often fell on environmental determinism to address the "inexplicable." In his description of everyday life at the military compound, Baily explained that many of the soldiers were falling sick for "no obvious medical reason." Baily wrote, that as early as June, servicemen presented with "Neurasthenia, headache, nervousness, sleeplessness, an inability to concentrate, and a constant habit of falling sick. In some extreme cases patients fell unconscious, turned blue in the face and ceased to breathe and often died in a few minutes."[31] Baily blamed the inexplicable breakdown of military bodies on the harsh environmental conditions in which the troops were trapped. Describing a hot summer day while at camp in the southern humid regions of Iraq, Baily wrote:

> A typical day at this season starts with a dawn which comes as a sudden yellow glare behind the motionless palms, lighting up a host of glittering dragon-flies, which rise out of the marshes and chase the mosquitoes. During the night the temperature would have been about 90 [Fahrenheit], and most of the time would have been spent in listening to the chorus of barking dogs, braying asses and crowing fowls from the village, the croaking of myriads of frogs from the creek, and the dismal wail of the jackal out on the desert.[32]

Baily doesn't waste the opportunity to express the sentiments of everyday despair and "fatalism" that he and the troops had endured:

> At noon, active work ceases, the thermometer being then about 115 degrees Ft. and the sun beats like a leaden club through the roofs of the tents, and silence falls on the scene. Any active exertion or mental worry at this time is intolerable. If a dripping orderly comes to rouse one to see some case, one can understand perfectly the frame of mind which has produced the idea of kismet. Why move? If the man dies it is the Will of Allah. It is the Will of Allah that he is sick. Let him remain in the hands

of Allah. . . . At about 5 p.m. the temperature falls, but the humidity rises and a period of the most extreme discomfort sets in. Even when sitting in one's tent, the clothes become wringing wet with perspiration. The few sparrows and blue Jays in the groves sit motionless, with their beaks wide open, panting for breath.[33]

For Baily, the consequences of the heat were only surpassed by the physical and mental effects of the Mesopotamian scenery on the servicemen. Describing the scenery on the outskirts of Baghdad where his compound was located, he wrote:

> The environs of Baghdad consist of arid and uninviting desert. On walking round the encircling mound, the predominant impression is one of death. The moat contains the carcasses and bones of dead animals, with kite Hawks hovering and calling overhead. At intervals are placed large numbers of Mohammedan graves. Every landmark is a tomb. On the southern boundary is the conical spire which marks the tomb of Zobeide, the wife of Haroun-al-Rachid, the hero of many of the tales of Arabian nights. Here the graves are clustered so thickly that there is not even room between them for a month-old child. And usually, as one looks, a little procession is bringing along yet another corpse for burial, not in the hallowed precincts of the tomb itself, but as near the dead queen as may be.[34]

This state of "death" contrasts with the soldiers' mental and physical experiences of the "monotony" of the landscape:

> They lived for months and years with nothing to look at but over-lasting flat dun-coloured desert, and muddy river with ugly little grey boats, rows of tents, sometimes with [the] addition of a few palm trees and huts built of mud. All these elements are shown in the model of Mesopotamian scene, and a fair idea can be gathered from it, of the deadly monotony of a walk along the river dykes, evening after evening. One never walked out into the desert, as there was nothing there to relieve the monotony at all. It was the luck of a few to possess a gun, or a launch or horse, some were fishermen, whilst to those fond of nature, the sparse green patches of herbage and even the desert itself, teemed with interest, but such persons account for barely a third of the community. Nevertheless the

commander who could arrange counter attractions for his men according to their liking, was responsible for a much diminished rate of sickness.[35]

Sinderson, too, had something to say about the relationship of scenery to the state of his mental well-being during the river journey. He wrote:

"To disparage scenery as quite flat" wrote G.K. Chesterton, "is, of course, like disparaging a swan as quite white, or an Italian sky as quite blue," for such it was to me, to describe the landscape. One phlegmatic N.C.O., commenting on the horizontality and bareness, described the view as "mile after mile of damn all, with a muddy river flowing down the middle."[36]

Descriptions of mental breakdown further echoed in talks of acclimatization to the Mesopotamian environment.[37] Concerns about adapting to the local environmental and health conditions echoed with the general state of uncertainty about the long-term commitment in the country. In a short essay published in a medical journal, Sinderson wrote:

Acclimatisation was to me a depressing experience as I endured three attacks of sandfly fever within eight weeks of our arrival. However, it must have been fairly complete as from that time until I left Iraq on retirement I was not away from duty on account of sickness for more than a month in all, and this as a result of a very mild pneumonia following the worst dust storm in anyone's memory, a very mild attack of flea-borne typhus after an unforgettable railway journey from Mosul in the height of summer, and benign terrain malaria.[38]

Empire's Therapeutic Promises

The British colonial experience in Mesopotamia was shaped by the empire's own disorderly conquest of the country during World War I. Such experiences were translated in the everyday medical realities of occupation and governance. Discourses about the paradoxes of Mesopotamian history and ecology attempted to make sense of the "hostilities" of Mesopotamia. The country's ecology, it was said, represented a challenge to earlier British attempts to navigate the Mesopotamian territories by river. British doctors mobilized tropes of tropical medicine to understand what many saw as the inexplicable breakdown of military bodies due to the harsh environment of the country's climate and landscapes. Claims about the "breakdown" of the body and mind reflected different concerns about the "stability" of colonizing projects and their administrative regimes. This is similar to what science historian Warwick Anderson has called "colonial pathologies." Such discourses of pathology captured the frailty of colonial order, at once defining the limits and instability of the colonial project and opening the door to the improvisation that shaped the British military occupation and attempts to transform Iraq into a viable state.

The future of the empire in the country remained unfathomable. Baily's final comments during his presentation at London's St George's Hospital captured such ambivalence. For Baily, the occupation of Mesopotamia would be justified only through the promises of a civilizing empire. Pondering the ruins of Ctesiphon and the troubled memories and experiences of the conquest, Baily offered a vision of a new world order in Mesopotamia.

> I am in doubt whether any individual, however much he may have detested that land, could have helped himself from wondering at times "what will this land be like in ten, forty, or hundred years' time?" As a reminder of the civilization of the past, there stands and perhaps will stand for all times, that somber ruin at Ctesiphon which, in loftiness and majesty surpasses all else in Mesopotamia of to-day. But as one is carried down the broad stream of the Tigris, and sees the changes which three years have wrought, the new cantonments, the cleansed cities, the docks, the vast host of shipping, and most important of all, the blossoming of the desert, acres of new cultivation and peaceful husbandmen, where once was barren waste, people with little village tribes, riven with fratricidal strife, seeing all these things one is led to marvel. . . . Is this the start of a new era, when the land of Iraq shall once more take her place amongst the countries of the world? . . . And is the day really so far distant, when the waters of the Tigris and Euphrates shall reflect again the splendor of buildings and gardens like paradise, surpassing even those of the king of Persia, Assyria and Babylon.

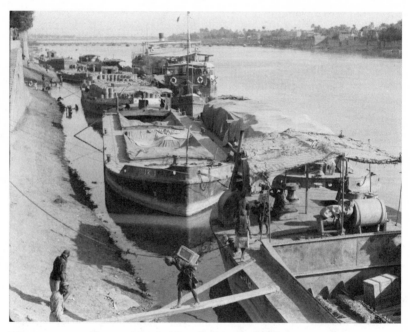

River steamers and barges along the Tigris banks in Baghdad, 1932.
Photograph by American Colony (Jerusalem), Photo Dept. Courtesy of the Library of Congress

2
Vitality of the State

Modernity is movement plus uncertainty.

Le Désordre, George Balandier, 1988[1]

THE NIGHT BEFORE British Indian troops entered Baghdad on March 11, 1917, the Ottoman military commander of the city left his post, taking with him the local police and officials and issuing orders for all records to be removed or destroyed. The King's Regiment, under the command of General Stanley Maude, faced no resistance as they marched at night into empty streets. Smoke was everywhere as the Ottoman army destroyed many government facilities and weaponry left behind. Less than one-third of the 170 Ottoman regional officials in the city remained at their posts. The rest either returned home or left the country with the retreating army.[2] Turkish hospitals were evacuated or destroyed, and the British found "only some few medical officers and some French nuns left in the Baghdad hospital."[3]

Addressing the inhabitants of Baghdad in his victory speech, Maude declared:

> Our military operations have as their object the defeat of the enemy, and the driving of him from these territories. In order to complete this task,

> I am charged with absolute and supreme control of all regions in which
> British troops operate; but our armies do not come into your cities and
> lands as conquerors or enemies but as liberators.[4]

A few months later, in efforts to reach out to the local population, Maude, in his first public appearance, attended an Arabic version
of *Hamlet* performed at the Jewish Community Alliance School. After
drinking contaminated milk served to him at the event, Maude came
down with cholera. He died a few days later and was buried in what
came to be known as *al-Maqbara al-Baritaniyyeh*, or the British cemetery, in Baghdad.

The death of Maude was metonymic of the medical dangers to
which no military rank or "supreme ruler" was immune. It highlighted
the risks of governing an occupation where contact with the general
population was becoming inevitable. Still, Maude's death was overshadowed by a larger crisis. The war had put Britain in financial troubles.[5]
The empire moved from being the main investor and creditor around
the world to the largest debtor.[6] Maintaining a full colonial administration of the three Ottoman provinces would come at a hefty cost, which
included managing the everyday threats of sickness and death.

There was no clear direction for Britain's postwar administrative
commitment in Mesopotamia over the long term.[7] The India Office and
Foreign Office in London disputed the semantics and configurations of
such commitment. India pressed to annex Mesopotamia outright with
minimal administrative control. The Foreign Office—under influence
from the Arab Bureau in Cairo[8] and British field officers such as Ger-
trude Bell and T. E. Lawrence—pushed for a form of "indirect" rule
such as existed in the imperial dominions of Canada and Australia.[9] The
United States pressured London to dismantle its colonial administration altogether and move toward President Woodrow Wilson's fourteen
points of "free trade," "democracy," and "self-determination." Across its
Iraqi territories, the indecisive, understaffed, and underfinanced British
occupation faced dissent and tribal unrest. Arab elites and tribal leaders
demanded that the British fulfill their wartime promises of independence.

The League of Nations Mandate reconciled Britain's concerns in
Mesopotamia with the prevailing international climate. In 1920, the

League declared Iraq a Class A mandate state under British control.[10] The Class A label signified that these ex-Ottoman territories needed "least" supervision. According to the declaration, these regions were deemed to "have reached a stage of development where their existence as independent nations can be provisionally recognized, subject to the rendering of administrative advice and assistance by a Mandatory until such time as they are able to stand alone."[11] Under this "conditional sovereignty," Britain's role was that of "trusteeship" and "tutelage" predicated on "obligations" to the local inhabitants while preparing them for full independence.

The declaration of the mandate was a great disappointment to some of the Indian government officers on the ground. At the same time, "the new policy was a welcome relief to the British Treasury after the high cost of the Mesopotamia campaign."[12]

Hakeem and Hakim

In the transition from occupation to mandate, Iraq became a site for "experimentation" in political and medical organization. British experience in the metropolis and in the colonies converged to shape the production of knowledge and governmental rationale of the new state in the face of emerging political, medical, and economic uncertainties. On the ground, epidemics and contact with the local population were real threats to the project. A few months after Maude's death, the Mesopotamian Expeditionary Force drafted "The Mesopotamian Civil Medical Services," a preliminary scheme for the future level of medical engagement in the three provinces.[13] The scheme was submitted to the Indian government. The opening paragraph read:

> It appears that the time has now come for some definite pronouncement regarding the liabilities to which we propose to commit ourselves in this country as far as the treatment and medical and sanitary supervision of the civilian population is concerned. . . . The great political asset of keeping in touch with the civilian population by means of medical aid has been recognized for some hundreds of years and one has but to read the great expansion of our Empire, especially in the East, to realize to some extent the predominance of the influence exercised by medical men.[14]

The scheme was ambitious and entailed a broad and expansive public health commitment far more than what military medicine and medical aid offered. It called for the extension of health care and services across the territories and proposed the expansion of quarantine stations, the development of a strict regime of health inspections, and a focus on disease prevention and reforming hygiene practices among the general population. These provisions went beyond the civil administration's limited national health care budget. The scheme also articulated the empire's distrust of the existing Ottoman health-care infrastructure and quarantine measures:

> The medical resources of the country are practically nonexistent. From extensive enquiries it appears that even at its best the standard of medical science and practice that existed before our occupation when judged by western methods was very low and would not have been tolerated in any educated community. The samples of Turkish medical art displayed by the medical men of the enemy captured from time to time could hardly be considered a safeguard or a trustworthy source of information.[15]

The scheme further emphasized the lack of local human resources and the "incompetence" of Ottoman-trained doctors:

> Attempts to obtain medical aid from the existing medical resources of the country were practically a complete failure. Even enemy prisoners—medical men—who volunteered to do civil practice and were accounted good, proved to be in the majority of cases very incompetent and were gradually removed.[16]

The report bore the fingerprints of two British doctors—Director of the Military Medical Services Colonel W. R. Battye and his assistant, Major Harry Sinderson, who had been seconded to the country's Medical Civil Administration. After the war ended, these two doctors strove to make sense of their careers in Mesopotamia. Sinderson had joined the war immediately after graduating medical school in Edinburgh. With opportunities in Britain uncertain, Mesopotamia was an occasion to round out his overseas experience and career in tropical medicine. Battye was a seasoned medical officer who had led the 108th Indian Field Ambulance Corps during Britain's failed 1915 campaign in Gully Beach.

Originally from Bristol, Battye was decorated for his service in colonial India's medical administration.

Undeterred by the financial restrictions, Battye insisted that the management of the Mesopotamian "ailments" required a serious medical commitment and expanded resources. In Sinderson's words, Battye was a "deeply religious man, convinced that divine purpose was the key to his appointment, [and] set about his task with astonishing zeal."[17] Battye's rationale was that focusing on medical organization would save the empire and its costly expenses from the present focus of providing limited medical aid.[18] He insisted that freshly recruited British doctors—preferably from Britain—should lead this new medical administration. In his autobiography, Sinderson wrote:

> Colonel Battye and I had long discussion with A.T. Wilson [Mesopotamia Civil Commissioner] . . . about the future policy, and in the course of it suggested that the new national organisation with which we were concerned should be called a Health Service in preference to a Medical Service. A Health Service was being promoted at home and we felt that in Mesopotamia there was even more reason to emphasize welfare in preference to treatment, which the word medical implied: prevention rather than cure. Much to our gratification, A.T., as he was known to his colleagues, welcomed the suggestion, adding that it would be an enormous advantage to the country if doctors could be persuaded to undertake political duties; the combination of *hakeem* [doctor] and *hakim* [ruler] was just what Mesopotamia needed, he averred.[19]

Wilson's clever pun on *hakeem* and *hakim*[20] resonated with strategies for a long-term commitment in Mesopotamia: if Mesopotamia were to be governed, it would be in the grip of a strong ruler and a wise doctor. Wilson's characterization spoke to his own approach to government. During his tenure as acting civil commissioner (1918–1920), Wilson insisted that Mesopotamia should be annexed and administered directly by Britain's government in India. He acquired the reputation of being stubborn and authoritarian—known among his rivals as the "Despot of Mess-Pot." Wilson had allegedly supervised the policing (and aerial bombardment) of Iraqi tribes during widespread protests against the British administration in 1920.[21] As a seasoned political officer in India, Wilson sought to establish an extensive administrative body to manage the territories. His commitment to administrative control was unflinching, as evidenced by his support for—and later, frustrated defense of—Battye's proposal in the face of limited support from India. Wilson's comment about the need for *hakeem* and *hakim* also invoked the broader debates in Britain about the role of doctors in government reforms of medical welfare. After World War II, such debates would coalesce in the inauguration of Britain's National Health Services.[22]

The debates in Britain about the stronger role of medical doctors in state organizations dates back to nineteenth-century European social medicine and political reform movements.[23] Political and medical reformers emphasized the state's responsibility for the health of its general population. They called for state institutions to play a more robust role in managing the growing number of industrial slums across Europe.[24] These reforms shaped the increasing appropriation of medicine in the administration of disease and illness in British industrial centers. Cholera and typhus epidemics among the working classes living in squalid conditions presented myriad challenges to government officials.[25] Cholera epidemics in particular hit hard in industrial settings, killing and incapacitating people and paralyzing economic production.[26] In Britain, the organization of public health further pushed state bureaucracy to expand welfare and oversee sanitary arrangements—vaccination campaigns and the provision of housing, clean water, and gas across the country. This shift was not only a strategy of risk aversion, but a mode of governance and state making in and of itself. As historian Dorothy Porter argues: "reducing the cost of destitution and poverty by preventing the premature mortality of breadwinners was one feature of a new theory of government which asserted that [economic] efficiency and justice could only be obtained through the scientific and rational organization of the affairs of state."[27]

By the end of the nineteenth century, state medicine as a mode of governance helped reduce the spread of epidemics in Europe. It also tightened the connections between state welfare and liberal economic practices that allowed for the continuation of production and commerce, and regulated movements of people and goods. The call for centralized, state-run health care in Britain enthusiastically picked up during the interwar period. Sinderson's allusions to this debate were accompanied by a sense of cautious optimism on the Mesopotamian front. Both Battye and Sinderson found in Mesopotamia a clean slate for experimenting with what they believed should be a stronger role for public health in shaping the future government of the territories. Iraq would be a laboratory for statecraft and improvisation to determine the limits of European health-care regimes. Unlike in Britain, there was "less" resistance from self-serving medical professionals and politicians. Both doctors also welcomed the opportunity to further their careers both as physicians and as political and social "reformers" who would take on the task of serving the empire through the uncertainties of the postwar period.

A series of political events and setbacks shaped the course of this ambitious project. Soon after the conclusion of the war in 1918, the government of India recalled its troops from Mesopotamia. Most of the medical personnel who were supposed to run the civil services were affiliated with the military. By the end of the war, up to two-thirds of the medical services staff had been demobilized back to India. The shortage of personnel and technical expertise undermined the civil administration in general. Wilson's main challenge was to convince the Indian government of the importance of medical organization in managing the occupation. Once again, the administration's ability to maintain order within Mesopotamia was in peril. In Wilson's words:

> [I]t is my duty to warn His Majesty's Government that unless they are prepared to grant the head of the civil administration in this country the discretion now asked for, it is not within my power to prevent a breakdown of the civil administration and of departments referred to immediately after if not before demobilisation.[28]

The response from India was not promising. It raised concerns regarding the potential financial burdens on the empire and the difficulty of deploying medical officers preparing to return to their civic duties. Postwar Britain's economic crisis, including inflation and increasing debt, was among the factors behind this ambivalence. Understanding the new financial realities, Wilson promised that expenses would be minimal and covered locally:

I am very appreciative of this urgent need for economy and of importance of not creating, as happened in South Africa after the war, a civil
service more expensive and elaborate than the country can hope to bear. I
am determined that no avoidable charge shall be placed on His Majesty's
Treasury even though some temporary loss of efficiency may result from a
policy of recruitment and modest beginnings, and I shall not fail to report
in detail all my proceedings in this matter.[29]

Wilson's reference to South Africa after the Second South African
(Boer) War (1897–1902) suggests an awareness of the burdens posed by
establishing an elaborate public health service that was economically
unmanageable and unpredictable.[30] Reassured by his awareness of the
need for financial discretion, the British Indian government approved
Wilson's request. He was instructed to establish a modest system supervised by British medical men and built with available local resources.
Only a handful of British doctors then serving in Mesopotamia were
ready to continue working for the civil administration. The rest were
either unwilling or obliged to return to their civilian posts. Knowing that
recruitment from India would pose a problem, Battye insisted that the
new recruits should come from the metropole, where doctors were less
tainted by the colonial administration in India and more supportive of
the need for an elaborated public health system.

During the summer of 1919, Battye traveled to London in search
of recruits for the newly envisaged health service. This turned out to be
more difficult than he had anticipated. Medical schools in the United
Kingdom were out for the summer, and he received no reply to a wire he
sent to the Sydney Medical School. Having to extend his stay in London
for a few more months, Battye circulated job advertisements in medical
journals with the aim of enticing both retired military doctors and young
graduates. Battye extended his stay for a whole year. His stay overlapped
with the finalization of the six-month negotiations in the Paris Peace
Conference in 1919, where Western leaders came together to decide on
the future of the defeated empires and their populations.

In April 1920 and during the San Remo meetings, the League of
Nations declared Iraq a state under British mandatory control. Protests
started in Baghdad and turned into armed revolts of different tribes in

the south of the country that took control of whole cities from the British military. With news spreading across the country, new revolts erupted across central and southern Iraq, all contesting British rule. The London government authorized the use of Iranian-based British airpower to bomb tribal strongholds in the south. The revolt ended in October 1920 with the surrender of the Shi'a holy cities of Karbala and Najaf to British authorities. More than 6,000 Iraqis were killed during these bloody months.[31] The rebellion cost Britain 40 million pounds and induced a serious rethinking of their strategies in Iraq. Facing criticism for his management of the rebellion, Wilson was honorably relieved from his duties as acting civil commissioner.[32] For unclear reasons, but probably because of his own reservations concerning the mandate and Wilson's sacking, Battye resigned his position and returned to India.

Although his loss was considered a major setback for the medical scheme,[33] by the end of that year he had managed to enlist forty-one persons for Iraq's new health service.[34] Sinderson and the handful of medical officers who decided to remain at their posts would be the "last men standing"—the core of British officials who shouldered the responsibility of engineering the mandate of Iraq's new health service.

Economics of Vitality and Waste

The declaration of the mandate signaled a shift in the British approach to health-care governance in Iraq. With the crowning of a new king and the establishment of a national government, the task of engineering the state was at hand. British advisers were assigned to each ministry, and Battye's recruits to the health service were now "gazetted" employees of the new Iraqi government. Attempts early on to create an independent Ministry of Health to run the proposed health service failed due to a lack of finances and staff. The reluctance of the British authorities to let go of the medical file completely may also have been a factor in this. The Directorate of Health was established as the official body under which health services were organized. It reported to the Iraqi Ministry of the Interior, which was more in tune with British interests at the time.[35] The role of the directorate would echo the relations between *hakeem* and *hakim* that Wilson advocated.

Both the Iraqi government and the mandate authority agreed on assigning an Iraqi medical professional to lead the efforts. Hanna Khayyat, a veteran of the Ottoman administration, became the head of the directorate. They saw him as a figure bridging the mounting tension between British and other local doctors who were close to the Iraqi elites.[36] Khayyat hailed from a Christian family in Mosul and was trained in medicine at Université Saint-Joseph, the French missionary school in Beirut. He had also received a diploma in forensic medicine from Paris. He was one of a handful of physicians of Iraqi origin who had administrative experience under Ottoman rule. He had worked for ten years as the head of the medical administration of Mosul's prison and its central hospital. Having "proper European" medical training and experience, he was respected by both British and Iraqi politicians.

Khayyat had a strong influence on the founding of the directorate. Still, most of the everyday work and reporting was the responsibility of the overwhelmingly British-trained staff. The directorate consisted of forty-four British medical officers, twenty-five nursing sisters, and twenty-five Ottoman-trained doctors. It also had close to thirty-two Indian and Iraqi assistant medical staff, including assistant and sub-assistant surgeons. These were distributed in hospitals and dispensaries in Baghdad, Mosul, and Basra, as well as in other "outstations" in Iraqi cities and towns. In addition to their medical duties, the role of doctors at the directorate was to regularly plot the progress, expansion, and challenges of medical and public health work across the country.[37] They submitted annual reports to the civil administration and recorded the country's vital statistics. These were further summarized and integrated in the yearly country reports submitted by the Civil Commissioner to the League of Nations marking Iraq's progress under the mandate.

In 1922, T. Barrett Heggs, Baghdad's health inspector and one of Battye's recruits, submitted the detailed annual health report to the mayor of Baghdad reporting on the expansion of public health in mandatory Iraq. In addition to reviewing the progress of public health work for the preceding year, the report laid down the principles and ethos of public health for the new Iraqi state. The language of the report had come a long way from the tropical medicine discourse of the war years. It resonated with the directorate's embrace of the state-making project in

Iraq. Debunking all the tropical clichés, the report sketched the ecologies of Iraq in a different fashion than the wartime portraits painted by medical officers. In the foreword to the report, Heggs wrote:

> Baghdad from the point of view of its prevailing diseases is not a tropical city. The number of tropical diseases in Baghdad is exceedingly small. A little malaria exists (17 deaths in 250,000 people in a year), dermal Leishmaniasis (Baghdad boils) is endemic, but also found in Southern Europe, bilharzia is occasionally found and is always imported from the Euphrates, dysentery is rapidly diminishing as a purer water supply is provided. No cholera exists; plague however, is endemic. The problems and work which face medical men here, whether clinical or administrative, do not differ widely from those in Europe. It is only a question of degree. . . . The mass of the disease is preventable.[38]

The analogy to Europe and the preventability of diseases were further emphasized in Heggs's description of the climate:

> The climate is not unhealthy. The sterilizing sun, the pure rivers, the dry atmosphere and the cool northerly breezes giving cool nights even in the summer, are natural features in favour of maintaining good health.[39]

Heggs removed Mesopotamia from the "tropics" to highlight the scale of the imagination of public health work in Baghdad that had once shaped cities in Europe:

> A sufficient and wholesome water supply, drainage and sewerage admitting of the abolition of universal cesspits, a good system of refuse collection and disposal, good methods of control of infectious disease, better ventilation of houses, less congestion of houses and more open spaces, less overcrowding of persons within the houses, better milk and food control and more arrangements for bringing good medical attention within the reach of the poor, are the public health requirements.[40]

Understanding that the difference between the work in Europe and Mesopotamia was an issue of finance and scale, he sketched the state's immediate and practical responsibilities in providing for the physical and moral well-being of citizens:

The prevention of all diseases is the duty of the state through its Public Health Authority. This includes not only epidemic and infectious diseases, but any disease causing mortality, suffering or financial loss to the citizen and so to the State. The prevention of disease cannot be divorced from the treatment of disease, for one of the best methods of preventing the spread of certain diseases is adequate and efficient treatment of the existing sufferers. This is particularly the case with tuberculosis, venereal diseases, malaria, bilharzia, dysentery, certain skin diseases and other infective and contagious disorders. In addition, in the matter of heredity many removable or preventable predispositions to disease can be avoided by the rectification of diseases and physical disabilities of the parent. The work of a Public Health Authority can logically be broadened to include all measures for the attainment of complete physical and moral well-being of all citizens and for the well-being of generations yet unborn. For practical purposes, however, it is desirable to concentrate public efforts upon the greatest evils and to combat the lesser evils as finance and opportunity allow.[41]

Heggs explained that physical and moral well-being were a means to achieving national productivity and averting "vital waste" to the state:

A glance at our mortality statistics will shew us much sickness and invalidity statistics will shew us more. Infectious disease statistics give one side of the picture. Hospital statistics give another. All this death, sickness and invalidity means waste. Waste of valuable lives and work to the State, waste of efficiency to the workshops, waste of efforts to the individual and waste or loss of money to all these. . . . Waste is uneconomic; it must be stopped.[42]

For Heggs, the optimistic, pragmatic reformer, the roots of waste were social and economic: "As usual, [in Mesopotamia] the greatest obstacle to the health reformer is lack of education and a low standard of living among the mass of the people."[43] Addressing the roots of illness entailed spelling out the state's obligations to administering the nation's health and the "moral" conduct of citizens.[44] Confident of the "progress" happening in Iraq, Heggs declared that: "A strong national revival is now taking place and a sense of public responsibility and of other proper duties of citizenship will follow. The will to better things is arriving.[45]

Departing from discursive determinism of tropical medicine, the directorate and its staff embraced a new ethos—one more reminiscent of the nineteenth-century public health reformers in Britain.[46] Heggs saw Mesopotamia with the eyes of a "bio-politician," and the biological and social conduct of its population as articulating the contours of the state and its vitality. This doctrine required that state "vitality"—the conduct of its citizens and economy—be maintained by eliminating potential waste. Waste translated as the loss of labor and disruption of economic transactions brought on by sickness and disease. Public health government was thus essentially a cultivation of the state by averting death and ailments at the social level. Heggs's "lesson" in state bio-economics spoke to the "survival" of the mandate state and the consolidation of its regime of governance. Its survival was implicit to Britain's aim to boost the empire's financial recovery.

Pilgrims in the Time of Cholera

The infrastructure of state "vitality" was already under construction by the early years of the mandate: the British had put Iraq on the fast track when it came to jump-starting the country's national economy. After the end of the war, trains, boats, and automobiles competed for the circulation of goods and people, and transformed mobility within and through the newly defined borders of the state. With improved river control, faster steamships navigated the waters of the Tigris, carrying passengers from Baghdad to Basra and back, and connected the country to India through maritime trading. Networks of roads and bridges expanded with thousands of motorcars moving across Iraq and to neighboring countries. With the motorcar, a typical trip from Baghdad to Tehran—which had taken three weeks to a month by the best available road transport—was reduced to four or five days at most. The British had begun enlarging the country's railroad networks expansively and had full control over its administration. Indian and Iraqi workers labored to lay down rail lines between Basra and Baghdad, passing through the town of Hillah along the

Euphrates. The British further extended the railway to the newly dis-covered oil-rich towns of Sharqat, seventy miles south of Mosul, and to Khanqin on the Iraqi-Persian border east of the capital. The railway carried passengers, goods, grains, oil, and military supplies across the country to its southern port. The British and later the Iraqi govern-ment completed the new line of the Orient Express, linking Baghdad to Europe through Istanbul. Advertisements for trains and railway travel to Iraq filled the walls of tourism companies in European and Indian cities. Travel posters portrayed Iraq's archeological sites in Ctesiphon and Baby-lon as tourist destinations and highlighted the newly compressed travel time between Iraq and Europe. Medical administration of the railways came under the jurisdiction of an independent department that reported to the Directorate of Health, and medical dispensaries were established along different rail lines.

While facilitating mobility and commerce, the change in condi-tions and technologies of transport engendered new "pathologies" for the directorate. The compression of distance and travel time was an express ride for vectors and carriers of disease. As noted previously, plague was endemic in Iraqi cities, and disease-bearing rats—lured to grain-stocked train cars—rode comfortably between different cities. The "unanticipated consequences"[47] of the rapid expansion of transportation infrastructure and movement were exemplified in the 1923 cholera epidemic, which coincided with the annual Shiʿa pilgrimage to holy sites in Iraq.

On August 3, 1923, three cases of cholera were reported among Indian workers living in a secluded camp on the river below Basra, employees of the British India Steam Navigation Company. *Vibrio chol-era*, the bacterium that causes the disease, usually spreads through con-taminated food and drinking water. It causes violent cramps, vomiting, and diarrhea with severe and rapid dehydration, and could sometimes lead to death in a matter of hours. In the camp, the epidemic escaped its containment, despite all the hygienic precautions. Five days later nineteen cases and seven deaths had been reported around the Basra municipality. Communication came from Mohammerah, about thirty miles south of Basra, that 133 cholera cases, resulting in 125 deaths, had occurred in Abadan, a town close to Mohammerah on the Persian side of Shatt al-ʿArab, where one of the Anglo-Persian Company's oil refineries was based. The directorate made arrangements to place a cordon between Abadan and Mohammerah[48] and Basra to prevent the epidemic from spreading across the border. Such measures were ineffective.

On August 13, 1923, the cholera outbreak was officially registered in Basra. By this time the directorate had attempted to put different measures in force in an attempt to control the outbreak, including stopping pilgrims from India and Iran; stopping third-class river or rail passengers to and from Basra; and requesting special passes from the medical officers of health in Basra from first- and second-class passengers; inspecting passengers arriving from Basra at all river or railway stations; and prohibiting the export of food liable to convey cholera from Basra.[49] The directorate also promptly opened a segregation camp at Baghdad's Quarantine Hospital to receive suspected cases from river steamers. Medical personnel were deployed along the traffic routes with the police authority to inspect all travelers and quarantine suspicious cases, but all measures failed to control the epidemic. Sanitation and quarantine strategies were not up to the new conditions of mobility and travel. Cholera cases were reported in all *liwa*'s (governorates) south of Baghdad. The threat to the capital was imminent.

Anxiety was widespread among British and Iraqi authorities. Later in September, on the 25th of the Muslim lunar month *Shawwal*, many Shi'ites made a pilgrimage to Karbala to mark the death of the sixth revered Imam, Ja'far al-Sadiq. Every year, tens of thousands of Shi'ites from Iraq, Iran, and India make annual pilgrimages to Karbala, Najaf, Baghdad, and Samara—a major source of income to the state and to the holy cities. To the directorate, the prospect of a tens-of-thousands-strong pilgrimage to Karbala moving into the heart of the epidemic was eerie. The projected magnitude of this particular epidemic was premised on the swiftness of visitors' movements as well as their numbers.

This was not Iraq's first large-scale cholera epidemic. The first major cholera epidemic was actually introduced into Mesopotamia through the military conquest of 1914–1917.[50] Since then, epidemics had come in waves once every three years, traveling along Iraq's ever-expanding commercial and transportation infrastructure. Prior to this recent epidemic, the British military had dealt with cholera outbreaks through the strategies of military medicine—to contain troops in cantonments under strict hygiene regulations. This time the case was different. The threat of the 1923 epidemic alarmed the understaffed directorate at another level: the country's existing quarantine system was obsolete in the face of the people's increasing mobility within and around the country. The need for new strategies for addressing epidemics—which would not only control the spread of disease but also preserve the economic "vitality of the new state"—were articulated in the directorate report on the epidemic:

> Infectious diseases in those days were mainly confined to local outbreaks, which when occurring in a large town, were sometimes of terrifying proportions, but which were shut off without great difficulties from other parts of the country by closing to all travelers the road and river routes through the infected area. Spread of disease by evasion of controls was slow, owing to the slow means of transport employed, and persons infected in one large town could with difficulty reach another large town before developing the disease. . . . The easy solution of preventing spread of infectious disease by complete closure of traffic routes was suitable to the Turkish administration, but can no longer be employed in a country which is rapidly developing and whose commerce, the motive power of its development, depends so vitally on the freedom of its traffic routes.[51]

For the directorate there was a political obstacle that needed to be addressed. Challenged by its own financial crisis, the Iraqi government had decided earlier that year to delegate central control of local dispensaries and hospitals to the provincial authorities. The main reasoning has been to reduce the central government's financial burden. Both the Directorate of Health and the officials from the Ministry of the Interior had strongly objected to such an undertaking. They had demanded that all of the country's hospitals and dispensaries be centralized under the control of the Ministry of the Interior, beneath the umbrella of the directorate. The directorate worried about the fragmentary control of public health that would result from this decentralization. Its demand was eventually challenged and rejected by the Iraqi cabinet, especially the prime minister and minister of finance.

With an epidemic spreading in Iraq's southern, predominately Shi'a cities, the directorate made a futile suggestion to forbid the pilgrimage for that year, warning of an imminent public health disaster.

Government officials, including the prime minister and the king, were reluctant to do so for fear of continued unrest in the south and the popular reaction of Iraq's Shi'a. As a compromise, the directorate received "carte blanche to adopt any measure of prevention, short of stopping the pilgrimage."[52] The directorate proposed to inoculate all pilgrims, travelers, and inhabitants of the two holy cities with an experimental cholera vaccine that had been developed in India. Experimental cholera vaccines had been reluctantly tested in India during the outbreak of 1894–1895.[53] At that time the Indian government, concerned with the effectiveness of the vaccine and the public reaction it might provoke, refused to make the vaccine mandatory for the general population.[54]

The directorate believed this was a good opportunity to test the vaccine in Iraq, especially after British doctors working in India attested to its potential success. The Iraqi government approved the mandatory vaccination proposed by the directorate as a more appropriate alternative to stopping the pilgrimage altogether. The production of the vaccine was beyond the capacity of the British Pasteur laboratory, which had been established during the war in the city of 'Amarah, so large quantities of the vaccine were flown in from India. Given the fact that the epidemic had already spread, it became apparent that such a supply would not suffice, so the directorate moved the laboratory from 'Amarah and expanded the central laboratory in Baghdad to manufacture large quantities of the vaccine locally. Strains were flown in, this time from Cairo—where a more elaborate and experienced Pasteur institute existed—and were isolated in Baghdad. The scale of the Baghdad laboratory production increased dramatically. The preparation of vaccines started at 2,000 doses a day and eventually reached 10,000 to 12,000 doses a day—enough, with the supply arriving from India, to meet requirements. As a result, two-thirds of the total 300,000 doses used were manufactured in Baghdad's central laboratory.

The experiment of managing the vaccination campaign during the pilgrimage represented a grave undertaking. Over the course of the epidemic, roughly 300,000 people—more than the inhabitants of the city of Baghdad—were vaccinated. About 90,000 people made the pilgrimage that year, and only a small percentage was spared inoculation. With the logistical and security support of the Ministry of the Interior, the directorate mobilized hospital and dispensary staff to carry out door-to-door inoculation in Karbala and Najaf—where three years earlier a rebellion was brutally suppressed. Inspections and inoculation posts were also established on all Euphrates crossing points, at Twairij, Musayyib, and Najaf. About 44,000 inoculations were performed at the Euphrates stations and in Karbala and Najaf, and a comparable number of pilgrims were inoculated at the Baghdad stations and in Samara. Vaccinated individuals were given a certificate. Any pilgrim who could not produce the certificate while passing any of these stations was required to take the vaccine.

The inoculation did not provoke any overt reaction, neither from the pilgrims nor from the Shi'a clergy—a success of which the directorate later boasted. The successful prevention of a medical and political crisis was further instrumentalized for political and scientific leverage. For the directorate, the management and coordination of the response to the epidemic supported its original argument against decentralizing public health administration in favor of complete central control over the country's medical institutions. *The Annual Administration Report of the Health Services for the Year 1923* claimed:

> The lesson of the utility of the various medical institutions in the Liwas afforded by the cholera epidemic was not lost upon the central administration and contributed greatly to the final decision of government to accept the maintenance of all these institutions. It is a consolidation for all the trouble experienced over the scheme to realize that the experiment has very clearly proved that municipalities and other local bodies in Iraq are not yet financially capable of maintaining adequate medical facilities for their areas.[55]

With the improvement in data collection techniques, the evidence of success was becoming easily translatable in statistical terms:

> The success of the preventive measures employed in this epidemic may best be judged by comparison with the epidemic at Abadan [in Iran]. Abadan, with a population not exceeding 6,000, had 961 cases reported, with 911 deaths (exceedingly high death-rate suggests a large number of unreported cases). Basra, with a population of over 50,000 had only 605 cases reported with 436 deaths, while the total of cases reported in the whole of Iraq were 1,640 with 1,100 deaths.[56]

For the directorate, the use of the experimental vaccine was an exercise in waste avoidance and cultivations of broader political authorities. The directorate demonstrated its capacity to become an efficient arm of government and security. The management of the epidemic also silenced the calls for decentralization of health care. It showed to the political elites the importance of centralizing and maintaining control over peripheral hospitals and medical units. That debate was finally settled.

The lack of resistance to the vaccine was also promising for the directorate. Unlike other experiences in the colonies, it demonstrated the extent of, and the tight links between, mandate and medical authority in the new state. For decades Hindu pilgrims and local governments in India had resisted the use of such experimental cholera vaccines.[57] In Iraq this did not happen. Ironically, decades later, cholera vaccines were proven to be ineffective and were abandoned completely by the medical community. Still, the enforcement of national public health regulations, and the ability to monitor new cases, was one of the main reasons the possible consequences of the epidemic were reduced.

The postwar political and economic crisis of empire set the path of British colonialism in Iraq. The reluctance to expand, the financial crisis, the role of global politics as channeled through the League of Nations, popular revolts, and demand for independence among many in the Arab elite all helped define the nature of mandatory rule. Concepts and experiences from the metropole and the colony faced new political realities. Exigencies on the ground required the development of an experimental regime of medical control to lead the country toward prosperity and progress. The cholera epidemic of 1923 was partly provoked by the rapid modernization practices and the transnational "movement" of goods, people, and technologies. The spread of the epidemic and responses to it also show the way colonial interventions could produce the pathologies they sought to avert. The responsibility of political and medical authorities had to be extended to manage their subjects' movements and conduct. Public health practices could "immunize" the state against the pathogens of development. As the next chapter will demonstrate, the biopolitical vision of *hakeem* and *hakim* became central to the state-building project.

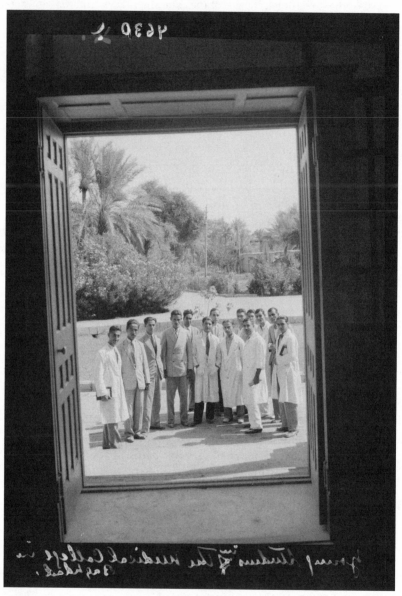

Students on the campus of the Baghdad Royal College of Medicine, 1932.
Photograph by American Colony (Jerusalem), Photo Dept. Courtesy of the Library of Congress

3

Doctors without Empires

THE POSTWAR CONTRACTION of the Ottoman state and its eventual dismemberment unleashed a commotion across the region. After the declaration of the mandate state, scores of medical professionals from Syria-Lebanon and Turkey converged on Iraq. Some followed King Faisal from Syria, where his short-lived Arab government had attracted a small nucleus of educated individuals from the Arab elite. Others had just finished their medical training or left their positions in the Ottoman administration to be part of Iraq's nation-building experiment. They followed the mobilization of other educated Arabs, such as teachers, invited by the Iraqi government to contribute to the expansion of the country's education system. Aware of the chronic shortage of physicians in this relatively neglected corner of the Ottoman Empire, many were lured by career prospects in the new state and the mandate's rapid modernization of infrastructure and services. Troubled by this unregulated surge of doctors from the region, the Directorate of Health attempted to channel the influx of doctors into positions in provincial and rural districts where the shortage of physicians was most acute. Many of the immigrant doctors disdained the directorate's efforts and refused these positions altogether. Instead, many opened private clinics in Baghdad, Mosul, and Basra.

In its annual report for the years 1919 and 1920, the directorate expressed its irritation with the "noncompliance" of these doctors:

[The number of local practitioners was] augmented during the year by immigrants from Syria and Constantinople for Civil or Military practice. They are, however, largely confined to the three big towns, and though in many cases keen on part-time institutional appointments in the three cities, they are as a rule, unwilling to accept posts as Civil Surgeons or Medical Officers in the Districts. It is a very great pity that this is so, as there is just as interesting a professional life in the Liwa headquarters with all its local interests as in the towns. It is difficult, therefore, to see how, in the future, such Liwa appointments are to be staffed without foreigners. British and Indian doctors in the Health Services have accepted services in such places, why not local doctors in greater numbers?[1]

The effort to cultivate Iraq's state medicine under the mandate confronted the realities of the transforming imperial landscapes in the region. The war had brought famine, epidemics, and the breakdown of medical structure across different Ottoman provinces.[2] It also led to the reconfiguration of scientific and institutional authority and with it the modes of professionalization for medical doctors hailing from the empire's former provinces.

As early as 1921, Iraq's doctors and political elites debated the need for a national medical school to train local physicians. Governing the health and conduct of the nation depended on the production of a state functionary that rose up to the aspirations of a modern nation-state—the *hakeem* and *hakim*. These debates laid the foundations for placing the Iraqi doctor at the center of national discourses. They also revealed the competing agendas, and overlap, of two regimes—that of science and that of political power—within the context of the region's political transformation. Iraq's scientific discourse and institutional training would be realigned to those of the British metropole. In this chapter I explore how such debates reflected the limits of colonial and national discourses about science and statecraft and disclosed the different forces at play in shaping Iraq's competing regimes of science patronage during the early years of the mandate.

Doctors from the Other Empire

One of the main features of the British Mandate in Iraq was the struggle to transform Ottoman institutional infrastructure and legacies.

Beyond being a form of masked colonialism, the mandate was a regime of political patronage aimed to reconfigure Ottoman territories in relationship to architectures of alternative political and economic regimes. Central to such efforts was the creation of a new network of "science patronage" that guaranteed the new nation's dependency on the mandatory power and its science and technology. This project refracted through prewar processes of change that played out in the medical field and transformed mandate-era political entities.

During the nineteenth century, the Ottoman state instigated wide-ranging institutional reforms to reorder the administration of its territories. This Tanzimat—literally "reorganization"—mainly came as a response to the rising threat of European powers and the upsurge of political and social dissent in the different provinces. The reforms aimed to keep pace with technological and military trends in Europe and to further integrate basic rights for the Ottoman state's different religious and ethnic communities.[3] The Tanzimat was predicated on implementing bureaucratic reorganization programs, as well as introducing European-modeled methods and technologies in the administration of the different facets of social life. These included, but were not limited to, reforms to taxation and land ownership laws, the regulation of military service, and the rewriting of criminal law based on the French penal code to guarantee the rights and freedoms of all Ottoman subjects. One of the primary dimensions of these reforms was the training of a new generation of civil servants to implement the Empire wide-ranging program of administrative reforms.[4] These included an overhaul of education curricula and training methods in schools, in particular the military where medical training of doctors took place.

Reforms of military medical education actually began a decade prior to the official declaration of the Tanzimat in 1839. In 1827, the Ottoman state inaugurated the Imperial Military College of Medicine in Istanbul. That same year, another military medical school was inaugurated in the Cairo province under the auspices of the Ottoman Wali Mohammed Ali Pasha.[5] In 1837, Ottoman officials established the Civilian Shahanian School of Medicine in Istanbul. In the beginning, these schools depended on the appropriation of European expertise and languages for medical education and training. The schools hired European doctors and adapted European curricula to train Ottoman physicians.[6] Ottoman schools also sent their graduates to Europe for further training in order to be exposed to advanced techniques in medicine and up-to-date medical training. In time, Ottoman doctors and students worked on translating French and German medical texts into Turkish.[7] In 1870, the Supreme Military Council made Turkish the official language of instruction. These military and civilian medical schools came to produce an elite community of physicians, pharmacists, and veterinarians who were crucial to the workings of the empire's expanding institutions. Doctors occupied important bureaucratic and administrative positions and were in charge of public health activities in different provinces that sought to make an impact beyond the empire's military establishment.[8-9]

The study of modern medicine was popularized during the Tanzimat. Muslim and non-Muslims alike were able to study medicine in the capital. In the Ottoman province of Syria, in the second half of the nineteenth-century, rival players arose to train local elites in science and medicine. The inauguration of two privately run missionary schools in Ottoman Beirut—the Syrian Protestant College in 1866 (later the American University of Beirut) and the Université Saint-Joseph in 1875—attracted local, mostly well-off Muslims, Christians, and Jews—men and women.[10] These institutions advanced the interest of the Protestant and Catholic missionaries in the region and challenged Ottoman hegemony in the production of doctors and other professionals.[11] In 1869, Istanbul introduced the Ottoman Education Law to regulate the professional practice of these doctors. Graduates from such medical schools were required to sit for the Turkish-language Ottoman Diploma Exam.[12] In an effort to further undermine these foreign-run medical schools, the Ottomans inaugurated a new medical school in Damascus in 1903. The school was geared to teaching modern Turkish medicine to Arabic-speaking students.

These doctors' loyalties to the imperial order were ambivalent at best. Graduates from the missionary-run medical schools developed diverse and mobile roles within these competing projects of empire and patronage in the region. Trained in English and French, many were fluent in both Arabic and Turkish. Through their relationship with Western education, some traveled to Europe and North America for postgraduate training. Others sought different medical careers in the Ottoman administration or military medical service. Although some opted to work as private practitioners in major cities or affiliated with local philanthropic institutions, many moved across the region to take up careers in the colonial operations of British or French military and medical organizations. Despite being confined to the junior ranks, their knowledge of the local language was a valuable resource for Western colonial doctors' interaction with the local populations.[13]

These regionally trained doctors were entangled in the transformation of the regional imperial order following the collapse of Ottoman authority. After the creation of the mandate, British officials in Iraq became concerned about the movement of Ottoman-trained doctors into Iraq. This was one of the main tensions refracting through the debates about the urgent need to create Iraq's first national medical school.

A Vital Matter

Although the Ottoman Syrian provinces had numerous medical schools, there were none in the three provinces of Ottoman Mesopotamia. During Ottoman rule the Mesopotamian provinces attracted, and depended upon, a wide range of medical professionals from across the region. During the Mesopotamian campaign, the terms *Turkish* and *local* doctors were interchangeable—mainly to refer to physicians serving in the Ottoman military and medical administration. As noted earlier, the British military insisted on excluding these "local" doctors. British physicians often criticized the lack of rigor in Ottoman medical science and training. The hope after the Mesopotamian scandal was that the supply of British and Indian medical personnel would be reinforced. The postwar shortage of medical doctors and the need to consolidate local health services under the mandate, however, imposed a new reality. There were only a handful of Iraqis who had been trained in the field—mainly as Ottoman army doctors.

After the declaration of the mandate, many of these doctors returned to Iraq to participate in the nation-building project. Along with British medical officers, they created a nucleus of medical professionals whose task was to respond to the country's immediate medical needs and to start to lay the foundations of Iraqi medicine. In 1920, these doctors created the Baghdad Medical Society (BMS). It met regularly to discuss a wide range of medical and health-related issues and to bring together doctors working in Baghdad. Discussions usually embraced an eclectic range of topics: alcoholism and its effect in Baghdad, the medical profession under the Abbasside, natural therapeutics, the demonstration of bloods in anemia, and tuberculosis in Baghdad.[14] The BMS would later constitute the foundations for Iraq's first medical association.

In September 1921, the BMS gathered for its regular monthly meeting at the city's British-built Quarantine Hospital. The forty-odd Baghdad physicians who attended had once been on opposing sides in the war. British and Indian doctors arrived in their military uniforms, while the rest showed up in Ottoman effendi-style suits. The latter were the "local" doctors—the term the British used to refer to those who were originally from Ottoman provinces or were trained in the Ottoman provincial medical schools. Two interpreters recorded and translated the transactions in both Arabic and English. Of diverse backgrounds—Arab, Turkish, and Persian—many of these Baghdad-area practitioners were not at all comfortable speaking English. Only nine of the doctors were born in Iraq. The majority communicated in Arabic and Turkish. Some had also studied medicine in French or German. Many had also served in the Ottoman military and worked as Ottoman health administrators prior to and during the war.

Iraq's general health inspector and BMS head, Major T. J. Hallinan, opened the meeting with a presentation on the health situation in the country using the newly collected vital statistics from the directorate. Hallinan gave an overview of the medical conditions and demonstrated how infectious diseases such as malaria, tuberculosis, and diarrheal diseases were still peaking across the country. He further highlighted how many of these problems were attributed to the shortage of doctors working for the Directorate of Health and explained the need to recruit more physicians to address that shortage. During discussions few local doctors proposed to recruit more regionally trained physicians to solve the problem. They pointed out that there had been an overflow of Arabic-speaking doctors from Syria, Lebanon, and Palestine graduating from medical schools in Beirut and Istanbul. These physicians were finding it difficult to land jobs after British and French forces supplanted the Ottoman administration of these provinces. The British doctors were uneasy with the idea. Responding to the heated discussion, Major T. B. Heggs gave an enthusiastic speech about the need for an "Iraqi medical school" that would supply "national doctors to deal with the high rates of local diseases and endemics plaguing the country."[15]

More debate ensued. British doctors enthusiastically welcomed the proposal. There was a clear split among the local doctors between enthusiasts and skeptics. Amin Ma'louf, King Faisal's personal physician, a doctor from Syria who had been appointed to head the medical unit of the newly established Iraqi army, expressed his excitement, stating: "The establishment of a school to teach medicine in the country is a form of economic and professional independence, which is as important as political independence."[16] In his turn, Harry Sinderson, who traveled from Hilla to attend the meeting, expressed his total support for an Iraqi medical college. He announced that this was an opportunity for "the recruitment of British academics and specialties, so far neglected and yet of immense significance for both the application of knowledge already acquired and investigations leading to further enlightenment."[17] Strong opposition emerged from a number of local doctors who saw in this project a recipe for failure and belligerent dismissal of regional physicians. Fai'q Shakir, an Ottoman-trained medical doctor from Baghdad, led the opposing camp. He believed that such a project could wait and that there should be no urgency in making such a decision. Responding to the unchecked enthusiasm of the others, Shakir explained that inaugurating a new medical school would incur a huge financial burden on the state and would be difficult to staff with competent local faculty due to the "shortage of qualified Arabic-speaking medical educators in the country."[18] Instead, he encouraged sending local candidates who showed an "aptitude for science" for training to Istanbul, Beirut, or even London or Edinburgh.

The debate was not resolved, and the BMS needed to come up with a decision on the issue. The doctors voted on the matter. To the dismay of Shakir and his colleagues, the British-dominated BMS voted for the urgent creation of the medical school. The BMS decided to act promptly. The doctors drafted a memo to the king requesting the Iraqi government's political, financial, and logistical support for the project. The opening of the memo read:

The preparation of means for the study of medicine in Iraq is an immediate popular demand and is a vital matter for Iraqis. . . . The government needs to take into consideration that establishing a medical college contributes to one of the most important educational branches, which leads to the progress and prosperity of the country.[19]

What started as a conversation about the shortage of doctors turned into a national debate about the nature and conditions of science and education in the foundation of the new Iraqi state. This debate further shaped the course of this project and revealed the dynamics and limits of the country's competing regimes of power.

Preparing the Nation

As a general policy, education occupied a low priority in Britain's colonies and received meager funding.[20] Authorities saw education as a luxury to which only a few select locals should have access.[21] In Iraq, the British feared that "by going too far too fast, a class of over-educated young people would be created for whom no employment opportunities would exist. Such young people would naturally come to form a nucleus group of political agitators."[22] Though both British and Iraqi elites strongly believed in modernizing and standardizing the country's education system, there was a deep divide in visions and trajectories of such an undertaking.[23] British educational experts frequently insisted on making English the national language for science pedagogy. These calls fueled anti-British sentiments because many among the educated elite believed that the Arabic language was central to the path and experience of modernization, a prerequisite for building modern citizenship.

The BMS call to create Iraq's national medical school was subsumed in these broader political and cultural debates. When news of the BMS memo and excerpts from the BMS meeting were published in the local newspapers, it stirred further debate among Iraq's educated elite. The arguments pivoted around the question of the "preparedness of the nation" for the study of medicine. Although opinions among these different voices were split on the subject, pressure on Faisal mounted to make a decision regarding its urgency. Sensing the political tension, Faisal decided to take his time in making his decision and to consult with his trusted advisers. For Faisal, this politically motivated decision was critical. He'd been brought to power through a controversial popular referendum orchestrated by the British.[24] He was coronated king in August—one month before he received the BMS request. Faisal "had to appear to be a 'nationalist' and not to be conforming to the broad wishes of the British government."[25] He had refused the original terms of the mandate that required his accession speech to declare "full subordination" to the high commissioner and the British government. In order to appear as though he wasn't under British control, he negotiated what became known as the Anglo-Iraqi Treaty, regulating British patronage in Iraq under the mandate.[26] Faisal turned to Sati' al-Husri for expert advice. Al-Husri had just arrived in Baghdad after being summoned by the king to take on the position of director-general of education.

Al-Husri was a cosmopolitan figure whose background, career, and movement embodied the complex terrain of Ottoman institutional networks of science, education, and administration. A well-known Ottoman educator, he later became one of the twentieth-century's main architects of Arab nationalism. He was born in Sanaa, Yemen, to a wealthy family, the son of a Yemen-based Ottoman bureaucrat from the Syrian city of Aleppo. Al-Husri studied history, French, mathematics, and natural sciences at the Mulkiye College in Istanbul—one of the capital's most prestigious vocational schools. After his graduation, he worked in a number of teaching and administrative jobs in Ottoman Epirus and Macedonia. During his tenure, he developed strong connections with the Young Turks—the political movement advocating social and political reforms in the empire. After the Young Turk Revolution in 1908, al-Husri was appointed director of the Teacher's Institute in Istanbul, where he led major reforms in the public education sector. He published textbooks in zoology, agriculture, and botany, which were taught in formal Ottoman schools.

Having been a strong advocate of Ottomanism, al-Husri was disillusioned by the allied occupation of Istanbul. He left the city in 1919 to join Faisal's short-lived Arab government in Damascus, where he was appointed as minister of education in charge of laying the groundwork for a national education system. After the declaration of the mandate, Syria officially fell under French control. The French expelled Faisal and his followers from Damascus, and in 1921 the British made him the new king of Iraq. That same year, Faisal once again invited al-Husri to serve as the director-general of education, this time in the newly established Iraqi Ministry of Education. His main task was overhauling the entire system of elementary and secondary education with an eye to creating a unified Arabic language program for the country's schools.

Al-Husri is among the most influential, and controversial, figures in the political and social history of Arab nationalist thought. He was a strong advocate of a secular model of education that could provide a common denominator for the modern Arab citizen. He saw common language and shared history as defining a nation. Everything else, including religion, geography, and economy, were secondary. His technocratic background, intellectual writings, and expertise were key in laying the ground for Arabic-language curricula and pedagogy across countries such as Iraq, Syria, and Egypt. During his brief tenure in Iraq's Ministry of Education (1922–1927), al-Husri shaped various education policies, introduced new teaching methods and curricula, and recruited many Arabic-speaking teachers and educators from the region.[27] Ironically, al-Husri spoke broken Arabic with a heavy Turkish accent—Turkish being his mother tongue.

Al-Husri was never at ease with Britain's role in Iraq and their interference in the education system—views that made him unpopular with the mandatory power. Many in the local elite resented him, even while respecting him, due to his somewhat rigid views about nationalism and his dismissal of the role of religion in modern education. Still, he was highly valued by Faisal, who depended on him in many decisions and gave him carte blanche to implement his ideas. The decision about the medical school was his first task after arrival in Iraq. In a book chronicling his time in Iraq, al-Husri explained:

> The idea of immediately "establishing a medical college" was one of the first matters that I had to look into and discuss during the first weeks of my arrival in Baghdad. The Iraqi doctors had consented that a medical college should be established without delay and the British doctors shared this opinion. The newspapers were taking notice of the idea and demanding action as soon as possible. . . . The doctors believed that since the hospital and faculty were available, it should be possible to establish the

medical college. Regrettably, they do not consider the *i'dad* [preparation/
preparedness] of students who would attend the college. . . . As for me, I
thought it was important to investigate this matter and ask the following
questions: How many high schools were there in Iraq and what was the
number of the students in these schools? And how many students graduated that year from these schools? And how many are expected to graduate
each year in the upcoming years? And what was the quality of education
at these schools—especially in the natural sciences? When I found the
answers to these questions, I became certain that the immediate establishment of a medical college was an erroneous decision. This project had to
be postponed for four to five years at least. At that time—in all parts of
Iraq—there were three high schools with four years education period not
divided into science and literary paths or specialties. The final year cohort
was not yet formed—except for one school that had only six students.
That said, the quality of teaching of the natural sciences at these schools
was very weak, mostly of an intermediate school instruction level.[28–29]

Convinced by this reasoning, Faisal delegated al-Husri to shape
the first principles of Iraq's education policy with the British adviser to
the Ministry of Education, Captain Jerome Farrell. An officer serving in
India prior to the war, Farrell was a strong believer in exporting British
morals and corporal discipline to peoples in the colonies. He held that
the "moral degeneration of the Iraqi people was due to vices of all kinds,"
and insisted on the value of "character building via cold showers and
team sports."[30] For Farrell, "[t]he best hope lies in the response which
the children have begun to give to the efforts of a few British masters and
three or four native assistants whom they have inspired."[31]

In his memoirs, al-Husri described Farrell as being very "rigid and
inflexible." The two men butted heads on several occasions concerning
education policies in the country. For two years, they relentlessly clashed
over the proper foundations of the education system in Iraq. In his
autobiography, al-Husri recounted one dialogue with Farrell, in which the
two "experts" discussed the language of instruction in Iraqi schools.

F: It is natural that Iraqi schools will not be based on either the Turkish or
the French systems, rather on the English one.

H: I agree with you that Iraqi schools should follow neither the Turkish nor the French systems. Yet, it should also not follow the English. I do believe that the educational system should be tied to the country's general conditions and its historical circumstances, and should not be transposed from another country.

I noticed that he was shocked with my comment, so I opted to elaborate.

H: I have no doubt that the current English system in England is giving fantastic results that no one can deny. However, we need to take into consideration that it is rooted in that country's values of family education, public education, and historic circumstances. If the educational system was deprived of this rooting and was imposed on another country with different conditions and circumstances, it cannot give the same results.

He then spoke about the problems with pedagogy of science in Arabic and the absence of scientific terms in the language.

H: This is not as grave a problem as you think. . . . The Turks teach sciences in Turkish, even in colleges of medicine, engineering, and agriculture; however, the terms that they use are actually Arabic in all the senses of the word. Even some of those who translated these terms are originally of Arab backgrounds. Take Basil Na'oum, for example, he translated the chemistry terminologies into Turkish. He is originally from Aleppo. . . . I don't see any problem with using the terms as is or with some modification; the most important aspect in my view is the language that is used in explaining and explicating.[32]

Al-Husri's vision of "preparing" the national doctor went beyond addressing immediate medical needs. At stake was the "formation of a citizen" minted through carefully crafted Arabic science curricula. Al-Husri recounted the conversation with Farrell about his decision to delay the establishment of the medical school:

F: You know that the decision about the medical college is going to be made in the next few days and I was told that you opposed the project. I wanted to know directly your thoughts about it.

I explained my opinion and why I had made my decision.

F: I totally agree with you that we need first to prepare secondary school education for that matter.

I was pleased to hear him say that. This was the first matter that we both agreed on. Yet, my joy did not last. I realized that what he meant by "preparing secondary school education" was making English the language of teaching for the natural sciences. . . . To emphasize my opinion, I reminded him: "Don't forget that the Arab revolution was levied on the Ottoman state so that more attention would be given to the Arabic language. Arab movements have started to demand that education should be in Arabic in primary and secondary schools. That is why we shouldn't think of introducing English as the language of sciences in secondary schools."

F: But these matters are only the concern of enlightened elites. As for the lay people, they really don't care about this a bit.

I objected strongly to what he said and told him.

H: Let me tell you that you are downright wrong. All people, regardless of their class, are concerned deeply with the Arabic language and I reemphasize that the Arab revolt was levied against the Ottoman state primarily because of concerns about the Arabic language. They allied with the British government for such a reason more than anything else. So it is not permissible to accept making the education of sciences in English, for whatever reason.[33]

These "expert" debates suggested that the interlocutors shared a vision to modernize state education—the preparation of students under a national curriculum. They also revealed the divergence of their political ends. Al-Husri informed the king of the details of his discussions with Farrell and convinced him to turn down the BMS initiative. In response to the BMS request, the king asked his head of court to write the following letter to explain his decision:

His Royal Highness has ordered me to inform you about the results of his inquiry. His Excellency shares with the BMS the importance and immediate need for establishing a medical college in the country; however, he believes that it is currently premature to think of this matter since the national levels of education are substandard to the extent that it would be difficult to prepare students with aptitude for this serious field of study. Thus, His Highness opts that his government would not institutionalize a medical college before working on improving the levels of education.[34]

Despite the disappointment of most BMS doctors, they accepted the king's decision, with reservations. For the next two years, Farrell and al-Husri continued to clash over many education-related subjects. Soon they were both out of the picture. Farrell resigned his post in 1922 and was transferred back to India.[35] For his part, al-Husri clashed with many members of the Iraqi elite. In 1927, he was demoted from his position as the director-general of education and was put in charge of the Iraqi Antiquities Museum. He held other positions until his final exile from Iraq in 1941. Although the project was not implemented at that time, the language of instruction was an issue that would haunt later efforts to create the medical school.

Who Is a Local Doctor?

Postponing the opening of the medical school had implications for the migration of physicians into Iraq. By 1923, al-Husri's policies and recruitment of Arabic-speaking teachers to the country's burgeoning school system had usurped British control over the education sector. The British-controlled Directorate of Health did not want to see this pattern repeated in the medical sector—health care having greater implications on British interests in Iraqi security and commerce. It hesitated to open the doors to non-Iraqi Arabic-speaking doctors for fear of being outnumbered by them, assuming they would take over leading roles in shaping the country's medical and public health policies. Keen to avoid a political crisis with the Iraqis, British officials at the directorate were also cautious of dismissing these doctors altogether. The directorate accepted the inadequate control over the "local" practitioners and allowed them to operate in cities and major towns. Although the small number of local doctors was still manageable, a few years later another political crisis compounded the strained relationship between the directorate and regionally trained doctors.

Mustafa Kemal Ataturk promulgated a new Turkish constitution in 1924, which effectively shut the new republic's borders to non-Turkish nationals, including erstwhile Ottoman citizens newly graduated from medical schools in Syria. Denied citizenship, many doctors of Arab origin thus had to leave Turkey, and over the next few years they began arriving in Iraq's main cities. This presented a further dilemma to the directorate. The annual health report from 1923–1924 raised concerns over the surge in the number of in-migrating medical practitioners. The report expressed concerns over using the term *local doctor* to depict efforts to "nationalize" the country's medical sector.

> The term "local doctor" is rather misleading, as of a total number of 102 non-British doctors practicing in 'Iraq, only 42 are of 'Iraq nationality, the remainder being Syrians, Turks, Armenians, Greek, Persians, etc. The Policy has been strictly followed to fill all Health Services posts with 'Iraq doctors whenever possible, and in Baghdad and Mosul the majority of the local doctors in the Health Services are of 'Iraq nationality.[36]

Sinderson, who was an important player in the directorate and one of Faisal's private physicians, explained his own response to the influx of regional doctors:

> There had been a considerable influx of private practitioners into the capital, mainly from Syria, during the previous two or three years, and their number was causing embarrassment, as many were finding it difficult to make a living. For political reasons the Government was hesitant to ban immigration from neighbouring states. The main trouble arose from the redundancy of medical schools in Syria. One or two of them were in name medical faculties of universities, and one at least nominally French, but competition to attract students was keen and rife, and in consequence standards were lowered and numbers of so-called doctors, far in excess of home demand, were granted licenses to practice. I paid courtesy calls on two of these institutions a few years later on my way to Syria. Evasive answers to questions and the little that I was permitted to see convinced me that there were grievous shortcomings in their curricula, and on my return to Baghdad I urged drastic restrictions."[37]

Sinderson's concerns echoed through Iraq's first national medical practice law in 1925. The royal decree gave the directorate the power to define and regulate medical practice and the licensing of "foreign physicians" who intended to work in the country. The law aimed to regulate the practice of all medical professions—including dentists, nurses, dressers, midwives, and inoculators. The law identified the doctor as "a person possessing a degree or diploma in medicine of a recognized authority, qualifying him to practise all branches of medicine."[38] A "recognized authority" was defined as "those universities, schools or corporations, having power to grant degrees or diplomas in all or any of the branches of medicine which the Directorate of Public Health may, from time to time, by notification in the Official Gazette recognise as a sufficient standard to qualify the holder to practise in 'Iraq."[39] The law identified a special registration process for those who did not carry Iraqi nationality and delegated the power to the Directorate of Health to issue and renew medical licensing and registration. Fees were due from all registered doctors. Doctors with Iraqi nationality paid 50 rupees whereas non-Iraqis paid 500 rupees. Non-Iraqi applicants also needed to submit personal documents and medical degrees to the directorate. The applicant would support the request with a letter from the representative of the Iraqi government in his own country indicating a clean criminal record, an authentication of his medical degree, and a testimony to his "good moral character."[40] In addition to attempting to regulate institutionally trained doctors, the law was a desperate attempt to control other "non-licensed" *hakeems*, including traditional healers, dressers (surgical nurses), and local *dayas* (midwives). Such local practitioners were integral to health-seeking practices in both urban and rural society. Most of the BMS debates concerned the higher infant and child mortality rates, which were attributed to the population's unhealthy and unsanitary social behavior and the "backward" practices of local midwives. The government campaigned to crack down on the city's "quack" doctors and healers. Many of their workplaces were sealed with red wax. The licensure law authorized the mandatory state not only to regulate the flow of doctors, but also to set new social conditions for medical practice in the country and to respond to the fractured national and imperial landscapes of science patronage. For graduates of regional medical schools, work opportunities in Iraq were restricted, lowering the curtain on the common practice of crossing Ottoman provincial borders for work.

The law signaled the revival of the new national medical school debate. In 1925, Iraq was declared a constitutional monarchy, and an Iraqi Chamber of Deputies was formed to function as the country's first parliament.[41] The election of the chamber was an important opportunity for the BMS to bring the medical school debate back to the political arena. During these years, the case against the government's decision to delay the formation of the national medical school intensified in the local press. BMS doctors were unrelentingly advocating for the school and the need to increase the number of national doctors. They wrote numerous op-ed pieces in the local press using the directorate's statistics on the looming threat of epidemics and high infant mortality rates as evidence of the pressing need for the medical school.

The BMS sent three Iraqi doctors to Britain to survey the educational curriculum in medical schools there.[42] This gesture emphasized the role of Iraqi doctors in the new college's teaching staff and the design of its curriculum. Simultaneously, British military authorities evacuated their sick from the al-Majidiyah hospital to the British Royal Air Force Hospital at Hinaidi military camp. This made the largest British military hospital in Baghdad available for civilian use. Its eventual appropriation as a teaching hospital was attached to the proposed College of Medicine. Al-Majidiyah hospital was renamed The Royal Hospital. BMS doctors used their political leverage to convince Faisal to approve the school. After intense deliberations in the Chamber of Deputies, the king approved the creation of the college in May 1927 and allocated 72,230 rupees—about $7,223—from the state budget to erect a new building and furnish it with up-to-date laboratories, equipment, and classrooms. For the directorate, this was the beginning of a new era, in which the erection of state medical infrastructure was possible.

The temporary shelving of the medical school and the ensuing debates revealed many of the deeper tensions running through the logic and practice of the mandate project. The exchanges within the BMS during the September meeting and the debate between al-Husri and Farrell over the language of instruction were not merely ideological in nature. At stake was the new state's infrastructure of science patronage, as well as its history, legacy, and future. These were further consolidated with the creation of the Royal College of Medicine, Iraq's first national medical school.

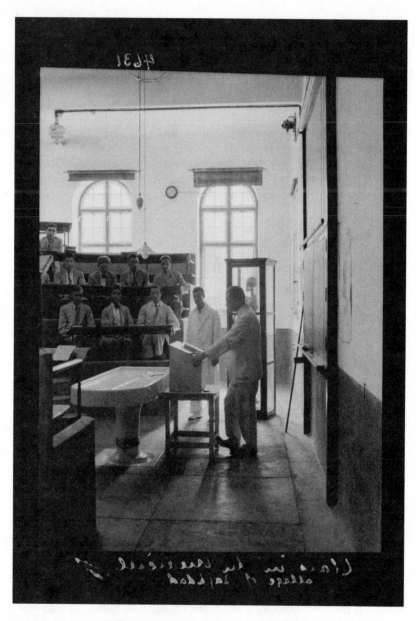

A class in session at the Baghdad Royal College of Medicine, 1932.
Photograph by American Colony (Jerusalem), Photo Dept. Courtesy of the Library of Congress

4

The Royal College

IN THE FALL OF 1930, the official home of the Baghdad Royal College of Medicine was completed. The inauguration was an official state event attended by the king, the British civil commissioner, government officials, doctors, diplomats, and other Iraqi notables. The Iraqi military band played the national anthem as Sinderson, the college's dean, handed the king a golden key to the school. Officials delivered speeches celebrating the school as a monument of modern science and education, and they praised the king for his undying support and leadership of the country. Located on the eastern bank of the Tigris, the building was strategically erected near the Baghdad Royal Hospital, previously known as al-Majidiyah. It occupied the northeast wing of the expanding hospital complex, which in turn expanded the structure of the hospital with new outpatient clinics, additional surgical wards, and a separate building for forensic medicine. Orbiting the main hospital building were the chemistry laboratory, the X-ray department, and the Pasteur Institute, which had been moved to Baghdad and expanded after the 1923 cholera epidemic. The building consisted of three large auditoriums, two lecture rooms, eleven state-of-the-art laboratories, a dissection room, a library, and three natural history museums that were furnished with myriad specimens donated by the Royal College of Medicine of Edinburgh. The pathway to the college was flanked by two thick rows of oleander trees, leading to a yard opening into the college's main gate. Two white busts of the Greek physician Hippocrates and the eleventh-century Muslim doctor and philosopher Ibn Sina decorated the entrance hallway—symbols of the Hellenic and Islamic genealogy of the school. Hanging above the gate a black sign, which read "Royal College of Medicine" in Arabic, was written in al-Thulth calligraphy.[1]

The medical school complex was far from isolated from its surroundings. It became part of a constellation of government structures expanding in the epicenter of the capital's Bab-al-Muadham district. To the north lay the cavalry barracks and the king's residence and, south of it, the army headquarters. The central prison and the state-run mental hospital were located to the east. The complex was positioned at the northern end of al-Rasheed Street—Baghdad's hub of commerce, small businesses, and coffee shops. Not far from the medical school was al-Midan Circle, one of Baghdad's oldest nightlife districts and bus connections. The medical complex was easily accessible to travelers from the rest of the country because it was located near Baghdad North Station—the capital's central rail terminus. People accessed the hospital from the other side of the river with small boats through *Shari'at al-Majidiyah*, one of the numerous riverside harbors extending across both sides of the Tigris.

In his yearly welcoming speech to students, Dean Sinderson often spoke to the cosmopolitan attributes of science in Islam and highlighted the kinship and institutional continuities between the Abbassid caliph Haroun al-Rasheed and King Faisal of Iraq—both allegedly descendants of the family of the prophet Mohammed:

> The first Arabic medical school was established by the caliph Haroun al-Rashid one thousand years ago. This caliph would be astonished and content to know that this college would be reestablished by one of his descendants, King Faisal, and to have as one of its first teachers a non-Muslim doctor whose name is Ibn Sinder (Sinder-Son)—as the first medical doctor in Haroun al-Rashid school was Ibn Bakhtyshu, who was also a non-Muslim doctor. For Haroun al-Rashid did not differentiate between a Muslim and non-Muslim doctor, only based on scientific merits.[2]

The construction of science and medical infrastructure at the college went hand in hand with state-making politics and the cultivation of British patronage via the mandate. At the college, the fashioning of doctors went beyond nurturing the authority of science within the walls of classrooms, laboratories, and clinics. Sinderson's comment evoked the ability of the "wise ruler" to transcend traditional social boundaries through his embrace of scientific truth. Such discourses captured the broader institutional struggle to foster the school's legitimacy as a nation-state-making project and a site for the production of the citizen-doctor.

Since the 1990s, more than a handful of autobiographies have documented the personal histories and experiences of Iraqi doctors and their medical training at the Royal College.[3] Written by Iraq's first generation of doctors, these accounts offer an insight into the Royal College's prosopography in the context of the broader social and political transformations in the country.[4] Written with attention to everyday encounters, these accounts disclose the kind of social exchanges and impasses that shaped newcomers' experiences at the college. Such accounts go beyond the discursive and disciplinary practices of the institution. They give life to the everyday negotiations of power relations and patronage that shaped this state-building project and extended beyond the college and its scientific mandate.

Makeshift Years

The operation of the Royal College in its first two years was improvised, to say the least. While on a trip to London during the spring of 1927, Harry Sinderson received an official telegram notifying him of his appointment as the dean of Iraq's first medical school. After deliberations with government officials in Baghdad, he ordered that instruction should start as soon as possible, even prior to the completion of the new building. The rundown huts near the Baghdad Royal Hospital would serve as makeshift classrooms. The sheds had been occupied by the British during the war and were abandoned after the military evacuated the hospital. On his way back to Iraq, he stopped at Edinburgh for a short visit to his alma mater to inquire about curricula and to rally support and donations for Baghdad's new Royal College.

Because very few Iraqi high school graduates had earned the academic prerequisites for medical school, one of the main challenges confronting the Royal College that first year was the shallow pool of "qualified" candidates.[5] The college appealed to a broad base of applicants. Through local newspaper advertisements and word of mouth, the school invited recent graduates to apply and even reached out to Iraqi students still in high school. It also accepted applications from employees working in the government sector who had a good knowledge and interest in the natural sciences.[6] Approximately eighty students applied to enroll. The school established a selection committee involving representatives from the college and the government. The committee was headed by Sinderson, and it included two of the school's faculty members and two officials from the *Ma'arif*, or Ministry of Education. They looked into the files of the potential students and developed "official" and "unofficial" criteria for admission based on interviews with the applicants. The main criterion was the student's command of the English language. The school had adopted the medical curriculum of the Edinburgh Royal College of Medicine and, except for one Iraqi faculty member, all six instructors hired to teach the first-year cohort were British. It was vital that students be able to navigate the course textbooks and comprehend and communicate with their Anglophone mentors. Unofficially, sons and kin of medical doctors and urban elites were preferred over others. These were thought to have an "environment that was conducive to medical education."[7] Emphasizing the ethnic and religious diversity of the school, the committee selected twenty students for the first year: eight Jews,[8] seven Muslims, and five Christians, mainly from elite urban families—the majority of whom had not completed the national baccalaureate exams.[9] In the second year, twenty-one students were admitted, only twelve of whom had finished their secondary education. The rest had to sit for an entrance exam designed by the committee. The entrance exam tested the applicants' general knowledge of science, but most of all their command of the English language.

While envisaged as a professionally run secular institution, the college was first declared a branch of another provisional project, the

University of Al al-Bayt (1924–1930).[10] The University of Al al-Bayt was originally designed to teach a unified curriculum of Sunni and Shi'a Shari'a (Islamic law).[11] It aimed to assemble "religious scholars from both sects to teach according to modern methods."[12] The University of Al al-Bayt eventually faced fundamental political hurdles over its teaching philosophy and administration.[13] In 1930, it was closed for good. After its closure, the medical school continued as a stand-alone college.[14]

The college's administration faced strong public criticism in the local newspapers. Critics questioned why, contrary to the government's insistence on prioritizing Arabic in the national curricula, the school would teach medicine in English. Critics also questioned the dismissal of the national exams in favor of selection criteria that promoted English-speaking students. Responding to such criticism's, the government cancelled the entrance exam and requested that the college amend its admission criteria to be aligned with the country's general and higher education laws. During the third year, new bylaws were introduced emphasizing school policies' compliance with state law. They stated that all students of the college should have finished their secondary education and taken the national exam before applying. That year, only four students were admitted to the college. Attempting to further calm critics and exemplify the scientific rigor of the school, Sinderson, with the help of other faculty members, launched *The Journal of the Royal Faculty of Medicine*—a bilingual publication that encouraged relevant research and essays from the faculty. The first issue of the journal included the text of the Royal *irada*, or decree, that established the school, along with its internal bylaws. In the published bylaws, it was clearly stated that the "language of instruction in the college is the Arabic language." This was provisional on the discretion of the deanery council that could opt to revert to English, in the event that Arabic-speaking faculty was unavailable. For the next few years, the decision to teach in Arabic continued to be suspended during the first deanery council meetings of the academic year.[15] By the time an all-Iraqi cadre had replaced the British faculty, English had become the lingua franca of medical training at the college. It eventually became the main language of instruction in all of Iraq's medical schools up until and including today.

Behind the Scenes

The college managed to overcome the political setbacks of the early makeshift years. Entry to the school came to be based on a merit system defined by the national baccalaureate exams. The school attracted many of the country's brightest students, hailing from different cities and regions. During the five-year medical training program, the college was a site for socializing doctors and fashioning their personal and collective conduct. In addition to their instruction in science, the administration also promoted the students' participation in physical and organizational activities. The tennis courts left by the British military were revived and opened to both faculty and students. Students were also encouraged to organize and elect colleagues who would represent them to the faculty—a practice that governed student-faculty organization at British medical schools. The school's administration reached out to both the public and private sectors and secured nominal awards from them to encourage the spirit of competition and excellence in the student body.[16] These were all seen as providing a "healthy social life for the students" and viewed as part of "the physical and mental preparation"[17] for this professional elite.

The school imposed a strict uniform upon students and faculty—the latter wore academic regalia when lecturing, while the former dressed in gray pants, white shirts, neckties, and blue blazers. Students wore black neckties decorated with red, green, and white ribbons—representing the Iraqi flag. Elsie Sinderson—the dean's wife—designed the college's unique shield-shaped escutcheon that was sewn into students' jackets. The design was composed of a blue Y-shaped figure, representing the three waterways of Iraq—the Tigris and Euphrates merging at Shatt al-'Arab. A serpent and an open book were engulfed by the two rivers and flanked by two Assyrian bulls. The throne of the monarchy sat on the crest of the shield. The tie and shield were both ordered from the United Kingdom and were required to be worn as part of the school uniform.

First year subjects included chemistry, physics, anatomy, and biology. Classes were set for seven hours per day except on Friday and Sunday—the Muslim and Christian holidays. Except for forensic medicine, which was taught during the third year, all classes were given in English.

During the first weeks of school, students in anatomy class read and paid attention to descriptions of the internal structures of the human body. The teacher used a live "specimen"—a thin custodian who worked at the college—to demonstrate the outlines of muscles and body areas. At the anatomy lab, students were given the opportunity to translate this book learning into empirical experience. The instructor divided each class into smaller groups, each in charge of a cadaver. Students' first encounter with cadavers provoked many anxieties. One former student's account described how the smell of formaldehyde and the sight of the tan-skinned cadaver on the dissecting table sent shivers up his spine.

Calming the students and the public took more than the assurances of Sinderson and his colleagues. Students' training involved the supervision of the king himself. Faisal attended graduation ceremonies and handed out diplomas to the graduating doctors. He also visited the school regularly during the academic year. His visits usually coincided with the first weeks of anatomy classes. For the students, the king's visit was "an encouragement for those who feared dead bodies."[18] One student recalled such a visit:

> The King entered the anatomy lab accompanied by Dean Sinderson. While stroking his goatee, the King slowly approached one of the dissection tables as one student stood next to the cadaver holding half a brain in his hand. Sinderson began explaining to the King: "This is the human brain, Your Highness, where bundles of nerves arrive delivering news from the rest of the body and take orders from it. . . ." Interrupting Sinderson's explications, the King moved to the next dissection table where I was standing with three of my colleagues. He asked my colleague, Kamal Nouriddine, in a Bedouin-accented English: "Do you like Anatomy?" Hesitantly, Kamal replied: "Yes Sir . . . I mean, Your Highness." The king laughed and patted Kamal on his shoulder.[19]

Sinderson's elucidation of the relationship between brain and body using simplistic political metaphors might have been too apparent for Faisal, who was more concerned with the general anxiety of the future doctors. For students, working on the dead—and the source of supply for these bodies—provoked many questions. Many were uncomfortable about popular stories in their hometowns about grave-robbing. Among the faculty, it was feared that this discomfort would create a public backlash. This problem was not unique to the Royal College, as the supply of bodies for dissection had haunted European and North American anatomy labs and medical schools for centuries.[20] Tales of body snatchers and grave diggers had scandalized nineteenth-century medical schools and ignited riots in places like Aberdeen and Edinburgh—Sinderson's hometown. Tainted by this history, the faculty was wary of reaction "against the possibility of Moslems' cadavers being dissected."[21] In order to avert public controversy, Sinderson and the faculty spread a rumor that "bodies would be imported from European countries."[22] For the students, the mystery of the imported cadavers was eventually solved as they realized that their anatomical specimens were in fact being brought in from the nearby hospital. One of the school's custodians, Mullah Khudhor, was instrumental in meeting the college's needs for cadavers.

Little is known about Mullah Khudhor, but various accounts and autobiographies of Iraqi doctors allow us to piece together his story. Khudhor was born in Baghdad in the late nineteenth century. He started his "career" as the Imam of a small masjid (mosque) attached to Baghdad's Ottoman-run Namiq Pasha Hospital. He slowly showed interest in medical work and was eventually appointed dresser (surgical nurse) in the New General Hospital established by the British in 1919. He was appointed to the forensic department, where he acquired invaluable experience in dissection. With the opening of the Royal College, Sa'ib Shawkat, the anatomy instructor, brought Mullah Khudhor to work as his laboratory assistant. Mullah Khudhor helped in the preparation of cadavers for dissection, showing great skill in preserving corpses and performing postmortems. His knowledge of dissection and technical skills were readily available to students who needed help at the lab.

Mullah Khudhor was characterized as "illiterate" by many of the doctors, though he insisted he could read and chant the Quran. Describing Mullah Khudhor, Sinderson wrote:

> The senior mortuary attendant of the hospital was a massive bearded Arab, known to all and sundry as Mullah. He was certainly not, as his sobriquet suggested, a Mohammedan learned in theology and law, but the

designation earned him considerable respect, and he was just the man needed behind the scenes in the anatomy department. Installed there, he was soon an expert at preserving bodies for dissection as he was in the performance of post-mortem laparotomies and trepanations. To see Mullah at work in the mortuary, knife in hand, was an unforgettable experience. His deftness and celerity, acquired after many years of practice, were quite remarkable, although his knowledge of morbid anatomy remained elementary, and he cut and carved corpses with ungloved hands, contemptuous of the countless microorganisms awaiting the chance of invasion of hand or finger through puncture, scratch or incision.[23]

As the man "behind the scenes," Mullah Khudhor was acknowledged by the dean's first-year report to the directorate for his role in "supporting students and providing excellent services to the College." The report continued:

As their first encounter with the profession, students entered into the anatomy laboratory with pale faces, struggling between the wisdom of their choice and fear of the profession. It was the sheer presence of the Mullah close to them, enough to re-establish the balance and fill them with more confidence in the future and security about the profession that they chose.[24]

Mullah Khudhor did not work alone. He was supported by a network of janitorial custodians. Shaba, Marougi, and Mullah Yousif served as cleaners, messengers, and assistants in the anatomy laboratory. Among themselves, they had developed a division of labor to manage the school's multiple and precarious needs. Mullah Khudhor collected the students' lab coats every Thursday and handed them to Marougi, who would take them home so his wife would wash them. They also collected the remains of bones and skulls, cleaned and boiled them to take off the remaining flesh, and spread them under the sun of the roof of the college for days so they would dry. These bones and skulls would be used later in the museum or as teaching specimens for the students in the anatomy laboratory. 'Abid, the Mullah's son, worked at the hospital as an ambulance driver. Through him, the school custodians were further connected to the hospital staff of dressers, orderlies, and nurses.

This custodian network had a crucial, though far less publicly visible, function in the college. They ensured the continuous supply of cadavers from the hospital without raising suspicions and objections. Unclaimed bodies of poor and mentally ill patients were sought out. As soon as a person died in the ward, the school custodians would immediately be notified about the possibility of a new cadaver from the hospital. Mullah Yousif would first discern the economic status of the family. Having ensured their inability to afford the burial, he would carry the corpse to the anatomy lab for preparation by Mullah Khudhor, Shaba, and Marougi. If it happened that the family returned to the hospital, they would be told that the body was buried "according to the Islamic Shari'a in a special undisclosed Hospital cemetery."[25]

The corpse would then be carried on a stretcher in a ritualistic fashion to be prepared for dissection across the street at the college's anatomy lab. The parody of mourning invoked local religious and grieving practices in Iraq and served as an abridged mourning ceremony in preparation for an "afterlife" in the anatomy lab:

> As Mullah Yousif approaches the College with his stretcher from the hospital, he begins lamenting the dead person with his sad and euphonic voice. He would stop sometimes on his way from the hospital to ritualistically beat his chest with both his hands in grief for the loss, yet of course he didn't even know the person. When he arrives to the College's entrance, his voice changed back to normal and he shouted at people to clear the way "for the courageous cavalier to welcome him to the Home of the Afterlife and its wide heavens." When Mullah Khudhor hears him, he comes out to receive the body . . . the Mullah regarded it as prudent to shave the hair of his acquisitions, and so ensure concealment of identity.[26]

At the Royal College, students were being trained to internalize modes of sociality that would prepare them for their professional lives as doctors. Many behind-the-scenes practices shaped the early years of the medical school and its production as a state science enterprise. In addition to the role of the king and British faculty, the contributions of the school's custodians showed how the construction of forms of knowledge and authority were further complicated by the limits of the institution and its ability to further appropriate "alternative" practices for the survival and continuation of the project. As the source of the cadavers became known among the students, the acquisition of dead bodies became more accepted. It was a shared secret that everybody kept out of fear of public backlash and as a pragmatic necessity.

The next sections explore the trajectories of three medical students during the formative years of the college. Their accounts show the broader mandate-era state socialization processes of which the Royal College was part. It is also evident that different ambivalences of conduct and power relations were enmeshed in everyday social intercourses inside the college and beyond.

Fashioning Conduct

In his four-volume autobiography, *Hadeeth al-Thamaneen* (A Conversation at Eighty), Kamal al-Samara'i (1912–1999) wrote at length about his experiences coming of age in Iraq and becoming one of Iraq's pioneer doctors in obstetrics and gynecology. His book was the first autobiographical record of the Royal College's early years from a student's perspective. The account chronicles his personal history from his early childhood through his adulthood and career working as a medical doctor for the Iraqi royal family and running one of the most famous private hospitals in the country.[27]

Al-Samara'i, who is known to the generations of Iraqi doctors as "sheikh of the doctors," was born in 1912 in the old city of Samara— some 120 kilometers north of Baghdad. He was the son of a middle-ranking Ottoman official. His father had fought alongside the Ottomans during World War I and was among several locals imprisoned and taken to Serampore in West Bengal. As a young boy, Kamal received religious schooling at the *kuttab* (Quran school), where he learned how to read and write. At the age of ten, he was admitted to Samara's first elementary school, which was teaching the newly created Arabic curriculum. After finishing his last year of elementary school, he traveled to Baghdad to take the national elementary exam that was offered exclusively at the capital. Like many other small towns in Iraq, Samara's education stopped at the elementary level. Students wishing to pursue state education often had to move to more central locations. Kamal's family then sent him to the town of Hilla, south of Baghdad, to continue his intermediate education. There, he stayed with his older brother, who was working for the government's postal service. After three years in the local school of Hilla, he moved to Baghdad to continue his secondary education at al-Thanawiyah al-Markaziyah, or the Central Secondary School. One of the country's most prestigious public schools, it was the place where many middle-class and elite families aspired to enroll their children. After finishing his national baccalaureate exams, Kamal applied for entry into the Royal College. He received a letter inviting him to sit for an interview.

Kamal al-Samara'i was admitted to the Royal College in 1932—the year of the official conclusion of the British Mandate. Al-Samara'i was ushered into the clerk's office where he submitted his application and was given paperwork to fill out. He was later sent to the office of the college's secretary—where a large portrait of King Faisal in his Bedouin attire hung behind the desk.[28] The following exchange took place:

> Your name is Kamal Tawfeeq Mohammed?
>
> Yes, my name is Kamal Tawfeeq Mohammed.
>
> From Samara?
>
> Yes, from Samara.
>
> Then it is Kamal Tawfeeq al Samara'i!
>
> Yes, Kamal Tawfeeq al Samara'i!
>
> Yes, that is better, do you agree to adding al-Samara'i to your name?
>
> Yes, I do.
>
> From now on your name is going to be under the letter "Seen" and not "Kaf" in the college records. . . .Your interview will be tomorrow, Monday, at 9 a.m.[29]

For many students like al-Samara'i, the college was a new and unfamiliar world whose hierarchies they had to navigate to learn its secrets, gestures, ways, and modes of being. Al-Samara'i explained that this was how he, unofficially, acquired his last name in professional and social circles. He clarified that throughout his precollege education, he was known in official Arabic state records by his "triple name": Kamal Taw-feeq Mohammed. He explained that eventually he went along with that name because it worked with the way the college's official records were kept, "the British way." Al-Samara'i further detailed, what seemed to him at the time, a disorderly and embarrassing encounter that captured his yet to be "reformed" conduct and character:

That Monday, a number of applicants were present at the college for their interviews. I knew two of them who were my colleagues from high school. When one of them came out of his interview, I rushed to him:

Who interviewed you?

An English man.

What did he ask you?

General questions.

General questions, like what?

For example, do you have a doctor in your family? Why do you want to study medicine? But his accent is somewhat incomprehensible.

When I heard his last sentence, my blood froze in my veins. Before inter-rogating him further, the secretary poked his head out of the office and gestured to me with his index finger. He ushered me in and opened another closed door next to his desk and asked me to go in. In that room I saw the small "English man" sitting behind his office. He asked me to sit down in a chair next to his desk. I saw him take a pen and scribble a num-ber on a piece of paper in front of him. He, then, turned to me: "This is my home phone. Would you mind calling my wife? I need to speak with her." A telephone! I thought to myself. I had never used a phone before in my life. Also I have neither spoken to an English woman face to face, mind you on the telephone.

I stared at the piece of paper for few seconds, then looked up at him with a dull smile. I explained that I did not know how to use a telephone. He smiled back and replied: "This is obvious."

He asked me: Why do I want to study medicine? I had expected this question. I was prepared. I told him that I wanted to serve patients, especially since in Iraq there were many sick people . . . etcetera . . . etcetera. He then asked about which branch of medicine I wanted to specialize in: "Internal Medicine or Surgery?" At the time, I did not know the difference between the two. I remained silent. He explained that in surgery patients are treated with cutting and suturing, while in internal medicine it is with drugs only. I told him that I preferred specializing in internal medicine. At some point, he decided to end the interview and thanked me. On my way out of his office, I heard him calling back. As I turned around, I heard him say with a strict tone: "Say Thank You My Son!"

I did not understood why he said that and left the room realizing that he did most of the talking during the interview.

Accounts like al-Samara'i's give us a vivid insight into the dynamics of institutional life at the college. They illustrate the back-and-forth exchanges and negotiations of gestures and disciplinary practices that shaped the everyday life of students hailing from different backgrounds. Incoming students were expected not only to absorb the scientific knowledge and practice of modern medicine, but also to engage with moral and professional worlds that prepared them to become future doctors. They were expected to be cosmopolitan and worldly and appreciative of the state's science enterprise and its British tutors. With English being the language of communication and training, the school further fortified the students' relationship with British institutions. In time, fewer Iraqi doctors spoke Turkish, or indeed any languages other than the two official languages of the state—Arabic and English.

. . .

Other accounts of Iraqi doctors of the Royal College further show how conduct at the college involved negotiating broader social boundaries, trends, and practices that colored the landscapes of Iraqi state education. In 2005, Saniha Amin Zaki, a retired Iraqi physician who lives in London, published her *Thikrayat Tabiba 'Iraqiyyah* (*Memoir of an Iraqi Woman Doctor*).[30] Her thick autobiography chronicled her life and career as one of Iraq's first female doctors and professors of pharmacology at the Royal College. Zaki was born in Baghdad in 1920 to a relatively well-off family of Kurdish, Turkmen, and Arab backgrounds. Both her father and grandfather had served as officers in the Ottoman army. After the Iraqi army was established in 1921, her father joined its ranks. He also served in the Ministry of Education before serving as a representative in the Iraqi parliament. His daughter Saniha and her sister Lam'an attended one of the handful of elementary schools for girls in the capital. Growing up, Zaki recalls, she had more literary inclinations. She attended the Central Secondary School for girls registering in the literary program because she was hoping to become a schoolteacher[31]—at the time, a socially prestigious government career for an educated woman. She explains how female education acquired great value in the reforms promoted by the king during the 1920s and 1930s. Elementary education became mandatory for both boys and girls. More and more families were sending their daughters to public schools. Women teachers were becoming the modern role model, the criteria for which, Zaki notes, included catching up to European standards of fashion, reading more, and earning salaries that were more comparable to those of their male counterparts. More than a dozen of these schoolteachers were daughters of well-off and well-known "respected families." Some had received their advanced training in Beirut and Paris.

When Saniha turned sixteen, a family friend, the acting dean at the time, suggested to her father that she should enroll in the medical school. He explained that the administration was attempting to recruit more females to study medicine at the college and that she should enroll immediately even though she had missed the first two weeks. She would be the first Muslim woman to study at the college. Like many women at the time, in public Zaki often wore an *abaya* (a traditional black cloak that Muslim women wear in Iraq) over her modern clothing. Her father, who had insisted on her wearing it since the age of thirteen, had no other option but to let her take off the *abaya* when on campus after the acting dean told him that "it would be impossible [for her to wear it there] given the nature of medical education at the school."[32]

Like other incoming female students, over the next four years she became accustomed to wearing her *abaya* only on the way to and from school. Zaki recalls how taking off the *abaya* was an impotent symbolic moment in her life. More women were appearing in public without it— as a sign of the influence of modern times. She explains that such a form of veiling was more of a social convention than a religious issue. In time these conventions became challenged under the fast pace of social and institutional change in the country. Conversation about taking off the *abaya* for good had come up often with her sister, Lam'an, who eventually followed her older sister to study at the Royal College. Neither dared to make the bold decision.

> I was in my last year of medical school, walking out of the College with my sister after the end of classes in the evening. We wore our *abaya*s and headed back home. While still in the vicinity of the school, we sensed a shadow of a tall man pacing behind us. It was Professor Sinderson. He approached us and in a fatherly manner put his hand on my shoulder and said: "You are both going to be doctors next year." I looked at him and said: "I will take it off!" We arrived home. I sat on the chair in our shared room and told my sister: "We will take it off tomorrow. . . . I will talk to father right now!" I then recounted to my father our incident with Dean Sinderson. He looked at me for a while and said nothing! I understood from his silence that he was in approval. I went back to our room and I told my sister with exuberance: "No *abaya* from now on!" The next day everyone was surprised. But after one year all the other Muslim students started taking it off uneventfully.[33]

Zaki offers a subtle account of how women of her social class negotiated competing forms of institutional authority that refracted through everyday life at the college and at home. Although she captures the importance of the medical school's formative years in shaping everyday modes of social conduct, she also demonstrates how transformations, such as those of dress code and other practices, were part of the broader processes of state socialization in which other Iraqi women served as role models. Although few Iraqi women were admitted to the college at the time, this would soon change with the rise of women's education in Iraq. In recent decades more women than men have been admitted to the college each year.

The Scramble for Doctors

The college graduated its first class in 1932, the final year of the British Mandate. That same year, the Royal College in Britain officially recognized the Royal College of Baghdad. Three members of that graduating class were sent to continue their medical training and specialization in London. The rest were offered positions in the capital's hospital. Enrollment at the college increased yearly. Upon graduation, doctors were ranked according to their grades and performance. Each year, the government would sponsor the top students for full scholarships in universities in the United Kingdom to acquire the basic science and clinical specialties, with the aim of having these doctors return to Iraq to man an all-Iraqi teaching faculty. The rest of the graduates were offered positions and allocated according to the needs of the directorate. By the mid-1940s, a total of 557 male and 48 female students had enrolled in the school, of whom 204 male and 8 female doctors had graduated.[34] The government had aimed to cultivate at least one doctor for every 3,000 citizens from the general population. It fell short of about 1,000 doctors to reach the national target.[35]

The fashioning of "science patronage" between Iraqi doctors and Britain extended beyond medical training inside Iraq. This had to be further reconciled with the government's need for more physicians to fulfill their duties as state doctors. A range of issues shaped the continuing shortage of doctors in government service. These were seen as pertaining to the "disobedience" of the doctors themselves. Incoming students signed contracts with the government, committing them to at least two years of state service. Many doctors were reluctant to fulfill these obligations. Because many doctors came from well-connected families with high social standing, they often mobilized these networks, using political leverage to evade their mandatory service. Those who had such connections sometimes opted to travel abroad for specialization at their own personal expense. Others negotiated their way out of government service and moved directly to private practice. Some who did not like their assignments used their leverage to relocate.

In 1941, the Directorate of Health was transferred to the auspices of the newly established Ministry of Social Affairs—signaling the end of its administrative affiliation with the Ministry of the Interior. In time, the new ministry became an important stakeholder in defining health and welfare policies in the country. Once again, Sinderson was assigned to the ministry as an expert.[36] Per his advice, the Ministry of Social Affairs aimed to further address the shortage of doctors by transferring "a certain number of young doctors for duty in out-stations."[37] Aiming for a long-term solution to the issue, the ministry, coordinating with the Royal College and the Ministry of Education, established new admission regulations. A quota system was introduced for students hailing from the country's underserved provinces.[38] The object was to "discourage the drift to Baghdad"[39] by accepting more students from these provinces. The measure proved shortsighted. It assumed that these doctors would want to return to their home regions to continue to pursue their careers. Sinderson found that the ministerial measure faced resistance from the doctors because "provincial appointment was unpopular, largely on account of poor amenities, and every effort was made by hook and crook to be exempted."[40] Many college graduates thus moved to the capital and other larger centers in search of better amenities and higher income and status.[41]

Successive deans of the college expressed their own frustration with the doctors' lack of enthusiasm for research, which was undermining the efforts of state making. Writing in 1944, Hashim al-Witri, one of the deans of the college, noted:

> At the present moment only four of the twenty teaching chairs at the College are filled by Iraqis, the balance being made up by nine British doctors, two Egyptians and five vacancies. It has been difficult to find students who are prepared to undertake research for its own sake, for in their eyes the only advantage such work has to offer is residence in

Baghdad. The position could be improved by better financial endowment of research subjects. This is the responsibility of the Faculty Council.[42]

An account by Dr. Yousef 'Aqrawi reflects upon the tensions arising from the doctors' studying abroad and their reluctance to do medical service in rural areas. 'Aqrawi was an Iraqi clinical pathologist who spent decades teaching at the Royal College. He hailed from a well-off Christian family who originally moved from Mosul to Baghdad in the early 1920s. His father imported tobacco and cigarettes—a booming business in Iraq at the time. His uncle Fathallah 'Aqrawi was one of the handful of Iraqi faculty at the Royal College, a specialist in dermatology. His family's connections among Baghdad's business and professional elite facilitated his access to good schooling and his eventual acceptance to the Royal College. His older brother Ghanim had enrolled in the college two years earlier. In a personal interview at his retirement home in London, 'Aqrawi explained how his professional trajectory was colored by the expectations from newly graduating doctors in the mid-1940s. 'Aqrawi recalled the anxiety that overcame him in deciding on the next step in his life after graduating from the school in 1945:

> The last thing I wanted to do was to waste my time and serve in the rural areas. I wanted to pursue specialization in Pathology in Britain. . . . My brother Ghanim was exempted from his rural service after being the top of his graduating class. He was appointed to do his clinical rotation in surgery at the Royal Hospital. . . . I wanted to study a field that no Iraqi has yet explored . . . a specialty both the College and the entire country lacked at the time.

The timing of 'Aqrawi's planned trip to the United Kingdom couldn't have been worse. With the eruption of World War II, the Iraqi government temporarily halted the foreign mission program. The government was also reluctant to issue passports for travel to Europe. The Ministry of Social Affairs refused 'Aqrawi's request and sent him a warning to report for duty. Insisting on his plan for travel, 'Aqrawi thought of pressuring Sinderson, who had just returned from a trip to the United States with the king and the regent. He thought that the dean might

make an exception for him through his leverage at the ministry. Sinderson made it clear to 'Aqrawi that he would not interfere to get him a
passport and travel permit. At the same time, he encouraged 'Aqrawi to
pursue his plans for specialization in Edinburgh—the dean's hometown
and alma mater. Having received an implicit green light from Sinderson,
'Aqrawi mobilized his *wasta*, or clout, to obtain a passport and financed
his own travel to Britain to pursue his specialty.

'Aqrawi's successful evasion of rural service and pursuit of
specialist study abroad is informative of the interplay of sociopolitical
dynamics and the dual logic of the national medical education policy.
Physicians were expected to occupy the roles of both specialist doctor—
who seeks to train at prestigious Western institutions—and general prac-
titioner—who would serve in the countryside. Although not necessarily
mutually exclusive, the tensions between these two trajectories of professionalization would continue to shape Iraqi doctors' career choices for
decades to come.

. . .

The creation of the Baghdad Royal College of Medicine in 1927
forged new geographies for medical professionalization and science
patronage in Iraq. In due time, it became the main national resource
for the training of doctors and the benchmark against which other local
and regional medical institutions were evaluated. The college was Iraq's
first medical sciences institution, and until the late 1950s, the sole medical school in the country devoted to the consolidation of Iraq's national
doctors. It envisioned the cultivation of a civilized modern citizen who
is cosmopolitan, Western oriented, and loyal to king and country. This
enlightened doctor would be predisposed to progress—having faith
in scientific truths and embracing modern technology. Trained in science, the doctor would be freed from "backward" beliefs, traditions, and
myths. The doctor would learn to respect the laws of the land and behave
with manners in tune with his or her status in a modern society. Incoming students received free education in return for their dedication to
work in government service after graduation. Working in the expanding
central government and health-care system, the doctor would learn to
embrace state bureaucracy and hierarchy, and he would participate in its

production and propagation. His duties were to heal the ailments in and of society, respond to medical crises, and spread the miracles of modern-day medicine to the general population. The doctor would aspire to become a pioneer—a better clinician, a better scientist, and a better citizen. Central to this project was the tensions between the doctors' career ambitions and the state's desire to manage their expertise. This conflict played out in the impasse reached in trying to balance the country's need for both academic and clinical specialists and "barefoot" doctors to extend national health care to the country's underserved populations. With the inauguration of nationwide state development projects that aimed to transform and engineer rural life, the doctor would become more essential than ever to the state.

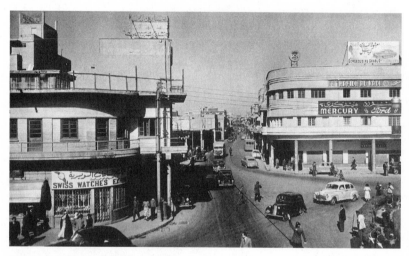

King Faisal II Street, Baghdad, Iraq, circa 1955.
Photograph by Ullstein Bild/The Image Works

5

Development and Its Discontents

> What is most important about a "development" project is not
> so much what it fails to do but what it achieves through its "side
> effects."
>
> James Ferguson, "The Anti-Politics Machine"[1]

IN A TALK delivered in March 1954 to the fourth UN Social
Welfare Seminar for Arab States held in Baghdad, Michael Critchley, a
professor of public health and social medicine at the Royal College, gave
an overview of workers' health situation in Iraq in the context of the
inauguration of Iraq's new development projects. Published as an essay in
a British medical journal a few years later, Critchley wrote:

> The biggest and most important industry in Iraq is undoubtedly agricul-
> ture, and great efforts are now being made to mechanize and to introduce
> modern methods of irrigation and fertilization. In England agriculture is
> one of the healthiest occupations but in Iraq it is the reverse. . . . It is not
> exaggerated to state that the average agricultural worker (fellah) is a living
> pathological specimen as he is probably a victim of ankylostomiasis, asca-
> riasis, malaria, bilharzia, trachoma, bejel, and possibly of tuberculosis also.
> If the various development schemes are allowed to proceed without the
> advice and whole hearted support and help of the public health specialists
> and sanitary engineers, such diseases as manmade malaria and bilharzia
> will spread to areas hitherto free, just as in Egypt.[2]

Critchley's invocations of the threats of the peasants' pathology
echoed earlier medical anxieties about Iraq's "tropical" ecology. As we
have seen earlier, the discourse of the abject countryside also featured

in Iraqi doctors' reluctance to accept work on the periphery on account of poor services and amenities. Critchley's comment, however, was not merely a medicalized representation of the peasant. He aimed to mobilize this discourse to point out the "iatrogenic" consequences— the "side effects"—of the development intervention itself. Across Iraq, development interventions were becoming imbricated in their own incongruities. Engineered wetlands and irrigation canals were turning into breeding grounds for waterborne diseases and increasing soil salination, thus rendering agricultural land uncultivable.[3] Development projects aiming to expand Iraq's cultivable land were causing what they aimed to control: the acceleration of rural migration to the capital. Tens of thousands of landless farmers were leaving their work in the countryside and heading toward the capital in search of better economic opportunities. They arrived on horse-drawn carriages and erected lodgings and informal settlements made of reeds and mud. They brought their livestock with them and sought work in menial jobs in the capital's booming modernization workshops. Critchley's warnings about the threat of rural pathologies captured the fears shared among development experts, government authorities, and "urban" inhabitants of the capital about the spread of disease and rural modes of life in Baghdad.

In this chapter I turn to Iraq's far-reaching development interventions and their "side effects" during the oil boom in the 1950s. During this period Iraq's statecraft was preoccupied with engineering economic growth and social change through development planning. Like similar planning regimes of the time, Iraq's development plans were predicated on accentuating the urban-rural dichotomy. In urban centers development entailed the expansion of administrative and service infrastructures, as well as the accommodation of the country's rising middle classes. In rural areas, development projects became more entangled in agricultural interventions concerned with expanding land for cultivation and mobilizing landless farmers to move to these new acreages. At the heart of this development dichotomy were lurking concerns about the modernization of the capital being undermined by unregulated migration to the capital from the countryside. Confronting their own limits, development plans were continuously being adjusted to respond to their own failings.

The shortcomings of developmental practices further produced broader discourses about the "incommensurability" of rural and urban modes of life. Narratives about peasants' pathological unruliness were not a product of development imperatives alone but part of broader social and intellectual articulations within Iraqi society. Such articulations of rural-urban clash and the state's attempts to respond to its own inadequacies metabolized in the legacies of al-Thawra City. Unveiled after the 1958 revolution overthrew the monarchy, this extensive social welfare housing project centered on one of Baghdad's largest informal settlements.

Iraq's Dual Organization

Sociological and developmental framings of Iraqi society have often been predicated on the tensions between urban and rural modes of social organization. This pervasive discourse was not imported; it has deep roots in "local knowledge" and intellectual production in Iraqi social science. In 1950, Iraqi sociologist Ali al-Wardi returned to Baghdad after finishing his government-funded doctoral studies at the University of Texas–Austin, in the United States. Upon his return, al-Wardi was charged with establishing the country's first department of sociology at the newly inaugurated University of Baghdad in 1951. He delivered a public lecture that laid the foundation for what is often termed an *Iraqi sociology*—an academic endeavor to use global and local theories of knowledge production to understand the "unique" social organization of Iraq.[4] The title of al-Wardi's lecture was *Shakhsiyyat al Fard al 'Iraqi* (The Nature of the Iraqi Personality). The talk was later expanded into a book entitled *Studies in the Nature of Iraqi Society*. Like many thinkers from the global south at the time, al-Wardi sought a marriage of Western theories with indigenous ones. In his work, al-Wardi juxtaposed the work of fourteenth-century Muslim sociologist Ibn Khaldoun on sedentary and nomadic social organizations with early twentieth-century writings on culture and personality—then prevalent in US sociology and anthropology.[5]

In his talk, al-Wardi outlined his analysis of the "cultural paradox" that shaped Iraqi society, in particular its ambivalenct relations with state authority. Al-Wardi proposed that one of the main explanations of this tension stemmed from internal clashes in the Iraqi psyche and between urban and tribal modes of sociality and values. Al-Wardi explained that, in Iraq, tribal or Bedouin culture valued *'asabiyya*, or loyalty to the clan, and had tendencies toward raiding. *'Asabiyya* encouraged tribe members to resist state control and to favor local forms of social cohesion. Under conditions of resource scarcity and harsh environment in the pastoral desert, a "love for raids and war," which brought the Bedouin a sense of "pride and heroism," developed as a survival strategy. On the other hand, urban organization celebrated docility and domestication, influenced by civilizational extensions of empires and governments into Iraqi cities. Sedentary city dwellers enjoyed a sense of docility that allowed political, social, and economic activities to flourish in urban centers under different regimes. The incommensurability of these two value systems and social forms contributed to what he deemed *'izdiwajiyat al-shakhsiyyah al-'Iraqiyyah*, or the "schism of the Iraqi personality."

For al-Wardi, this "dual organization" was not an outcome of primitive psychological structures. Building on the work of sociologists such as Max Weber, al-Wardi argued that the working of this schism is dynamic and accounts for historical processes that shaped the deep formations of the Iraqi "ideal type." He explained that *'asabiyya* began to figure in rural organizations as tribes settled in agricultural regions. In time, it became co-constitutive of urban life through the historical waves of tribal raiding and migration to urban centers. This "schism" was articulated during the alternating eras of war and peace that shaped centuries of Iraq's history. For al-Wardi, the dynamic interplay of these values guaranteed survival in harsh environments and in times of political instability during the historical encounters with occupiers and invaders.[6] He noted that sedentary values prevailed during times of prosperity. In times of crises, Iraqi society reverted to the tribal values of *'asabiyya* and war.

For al-Wardi, "social schism" represented the underlying "symptom" of Iraq's contemporary state-building problems. This "symptom," he explained, "has challenged the sociologists who have failed to diagnose Iraq's social ailments. . . . It is in this difficult phase that we are going through today that we need to understand the psychology of the

Iraqi people and how the personality of the individual emerges in it, so that we know how to govern him first, and how to guide him through new fields of life."[7]

At the time, al-Wardi's thought was far reaching among educated Iraqis of different social backgrounds. His writings engaged substantial scholarly work in both Arabic and English. His historical accounts were colored with popular ethnographic vignettes and stories from everyday encounters in streets and coffee shops. His accessible and playful writing style made him one of the most popular if controversial Iraqi public intellectuals of his time. His analysis of the nature of the Iraqi personality continues to be widely read and debated among the country's different social classes and has been commented on by generations of Iraqi social scientists and intellectuals.[8] The wide reception of his work and its recent revival in intellectual and popular articulations since the 2003 occupation, and his translation then to the English language by the US military, goes far to show the centrality of his "ungovernability" thesis to contemporary discourses about Iraqi society.[9]

Al-Wardi's symptomatology of social organization in Iraq might be somewhat dated and simplistic for present-day social theories.[10] However, his writings emerged at an important historical juncture in Iraq, marked by the embrace of state-administered, nationwide development and attempts to engineer the country's social fabric. His insights into rural-urban schisms might as easily be addressing the incommensurability of modernization practices that aimed to produce and respond to the dual logic of rural and urban development in Iraq.[11] His thought particularly reflected how the rural-urban dichotomy discourse failed to fathom its own shortcomings and the complexities of these two constructs in Iraq's history.

The Urge to Develop

Like many postcolonial development experiments, Iraq's social engineering projects were built on narrow concepts, (explicit or implicit) political agendas, and internal contradictions and paradoxes. As noted, the decision to expand the Iraqi state's economic productivity could be traced back to the postwar financial crisis. This compelled British and Iraqi government efforts to expand the country's commercial and transportation infrastructure and respond to the threats of manmade epidemics, such as cholera. The threat of social and political instability continued to preoccupy these powers after the mandate ended. During this period Iraq witnessed a number of upheavals protesting the policies of the British-backed regime. These expressed themselves in the rise of antimonarchy sentiments and the intensification of dissident voices, both in the discourse of the political opposition and in popular social mobilization.[12] Such tensions became apparent during World War II.

In 1941, a short-lived military coup provoked the flight of the royal family and loyalist political elites from the country. The coup was led by Rasheed 'Ali al-Gaylani and three other Iraqi army officers known to be sympathetic to Germany. The four officers objected to the Iraqi government's decision to side with the British in the war. On April 1, 1941, the officers mobilized army brigades to overthrow the government of Regent Abdulilah and the cabinet of Prime Minister Nuri al-Sa'id. Al-Gaylani was installed as Iraq's new prime minister. The coup did not last more than a month. Soon the British landed troops to occupy Iraq once again. Through its superior airpower, it pursued Iraqi military forces, forced the officers to escape to Turkey, and managed to defeat the coup. The British restored the regent and the government of Nuri al-Sa'id to power.

The second British occupation of Iraq continued until 1947, and with its end came promises of wide social and economic reforms that would bring a new era of political stability to the country. By the mid-1940s Iraq had already negotiated a loan from the International Bank of Reconstruction and Development for the construction of a large artificial lake north of Baghdad. The project aimed to expand irrigation to promote cultivation, as well as to control the seasonal floods of the Tigris. The embrace of reform was also a response to British and Iraqi governments' fears of Soviet influence among educated Iraqis and the country's disenfranchised, who were joining the ranks of the rapidly growing Iraqi communist party.[13]

Nationwide development plans and reforms proliferated after Prime Minister Nuri al-Sa'id negotiated a new treaty with the British government. The treaty dramatically increased royalties owed to the Iraqi state by the British-run Iraqi Petroleum Company (IPC) from less than 5 percent to 50 percent. State oil revenues increased from 3.3 million Iraqi dinars in 1949 to 50 million Iraqi dinars in 1953. Upon the recommendation of experts from the International Bank of Reconstruction and Development, the Iraqi government created the Development and Reconstruction Board (DRB)—a quasi-governmental body charged with overseeing the planning and execution of Iraq's nationwide modernization and development projects.

The board was constituted of both Iraqi and Western experts and technocrats who sought to cultivate new means of economic productivity and introduce social policies to improve the welfare of the troubled nation. It contracted international companies and invited world-renowned architects and development experts to participate in devising these nationwide plans.[14] The plans were predicated on three interconnected trajectories: the accommodation of the rising urban population, especially government employees and the emerging professional classes; the expansion of agricultural productivity through large-scale irrigation and cultivation projects; and the laying of a countrywide infrastructure of roads and services to connect the capital and major cities to the country's periphery. Less funding was allocated to the expansion of the country's modest industrial sector.

As part of these infrastructure schemes, the state invested in building local expertise in different fields of science, engineering, and technology. Facilitated by its patron-client relationship, the Iraqi state turned to Britain to build its cadre of national academics, professionals, and government employees. The shortage of expertise in these fields and higher educational institutions triggered a massive study abroad program, *Nidham al-Bi'that*—or Foreign Mission Program (FMP). The program was very much tied to the broader developmental fervor in the country. The government invested millions of dollars in the form of tuition fees and monthly stipends to support this program. It offered scholarships to students to study abroad and channeled them to earmarked specialties. The majority of these scholarships supported higher education in the United Kingdom and the United States. Such scholarships were also available from the British council in Iraq and other British/Iraqi-owned enterprises, such as the IPC. The latter were earmarked for the development of expertise in certain oil-related fields in return for a secure employment with the company.

The FMP was a merit-based system. Scholarships from Iraqi ministries were offered to high-achieving students who scored well on the national baccalaureate exams and went on to receive further training in science and technology, agriculture, engineering, medicine, physics, and chemistry, as well as advanced military sciences. Students received full salaries from the government and reported regularly to the Iraqi embassy. The expectation was that graduates would return and take on positions in the different Iraqi ministries or educational institutes, and participate in the management and maintenance of state-run development projects. Although some opted to stay in the United Kingdom for different political or career-related reasons, the majority returned. Those who returned received many social privileges from the state, including a well-paid government job, discounted lots of land, and loans to build their homes in the capital or other major cities. The return of these experts from abroad represented an important asset for the state. In addition to the large number of professionals graduating from Iraqi educational institutes, these men and women would form the nucleus of a national professional and middle class—Iraq's new urban middle class. Many of these experts would move across the country working on different projects and in various government sectors. Over the next decade, hundreds of Iraqis of different backgrounds received their undergraduate and postgraduate education in the West, and their expertise became integral to the state's development and administrative infrastructure.

The main focus of economic development was boosting the agricultural sector. One of the tasks of the DRB was to mobilize the country's underutilized natural resources by expanding and modernizing agricultural practices. These large-scale agricultural reforms were premised on the expansion of land cultivation through the introduction of dams, irrigation canals, and reservoirs to control river flows and make barren land arable. These interventions aimed further to counter the growing problem of rural-urban migration. According to the census, the rural population was declining rapidly. Between 1932 and 1952, the portion of the national population living in the countryside had dropped from

70 percent to 53 percent.[15] Every year farmers abandoned their land, driven by irrigation irregularities and exploitation by their sheikhs under the *'iqta'* system of sharecropping and agricultural tenancy.[16]

The rural development proposals assumed that by providing new, state-controlled acreage, landless farmers would take advantage of the opportunity and move in. Providing land was linked to another "natural" problem, that is, unchecked seasonal floods. The inundated Tigris had a history of causing carnage to crops on both public and private properties, thus creating the appropriate conditions for the spread of disease. The flood of the Tigris mainly affected the south, which contributed to farmers' seasonal, and permanent, migration from the land.

Echoing the early British preoccupation with the unruliness of the rivers for navigation, the "technical fixes" for agriculture focused on reining in the rivers.[17] As one report argued: "The two great rivers, the Tigris and the Euphrates, which constitute the framework and foundation of Iraq's life, are temperamental and difficult to control."[18] In 1952, work started on the construction of two major reservoirs intended to channel the overflow during the rivers' flood seasons. The creation of the lakes and canals was aimed at extending irrigation and to develop state-run agricultural resettlement projects. The largest of these were in the Dujaila and Musayyib regions, where the state offered landless farming families the option of either owning or renting land from it. In return, the farmer would commit to living with his family on the plot. Applicants from Kut and 'Amarah, the two cities where the project was located, were given priority. The hope was that impoverished farmers from these regions, who constituted the largest number of migrants to the capital, would move to such lots.

The technical language describing these new government-owned agricultural projects masked the state's deep desire to weaken the authority of the tribal lords and recast rural society. In development reports, the tribal sheikh was cast "implicitly or explicitly in the devil's role as the stumbling block to progress, the exploiter of the poor, and the general robber baron of the piece."[19] At the same time, the pro-British government demonstrated little will to directly undermine the rural notables' authority. The "feudal sheikh," or "tribal lord," was central to the foundations of the mandate's political system. Many were active members of parliament—by the British installed there as brokers of political security in the countryside. They had managed to advance their economic interests by acting as both agitators and peace proxies for the British and the Iraqi government, whose interest was to maintain a sense of security in the tribal-controlled areas.[20]

Although the state was unwilling to undermine tribal authority directly, it did aim to create an alternative space for negotiating new forms of rural sociality. The settlement projects in Dujaila and Musayyib aimed to transform the farmer's "tribal ties" in favor of creating small "nuclear families" that would mix with other families in the formation of the social fabric of these settlements. As one account explained: "Great care was taken to settle people of different local tribes adjacent to each other so as to promote amalgamation and hence long range community harmony."[21]

According to anthropologist Robert Fernea, who conducted fieldwork in the south of Iraq during the late 1950s, these projects' misconceptions included a narrow Eurocentric understanding of the notion of the family:

> Not only will this hypothetical family contribute to increased agricultural production, but it is assumed it will also help constitute a new social class, more interested in the development of community and country, less bound by tradition—the backbone of a modern democratic society.[22]

Fernea continued:

> While . . . the . . . experts were notably astute in much of their analysis of the contemporary scene, their estimation of the *difference* which agrarian reform would make was, one infers, based on the assumption that once given his own land, the Iraqi cultivator would take up his shovel and spade with the industry and attitudes of any proper English—or American—freeholder.[23]

Amid these short-sighted inferences, veiled political intentions, and developmental shortcomings, migration to Baghdad did not relent. Efforts to modernize urban infrastructure continued to face the social and medical problems associated with rural in-migration.

Dynapolis

The mandate's elevation of Baghdad as the administrative center of the state brought new social realities to the city and its residents. Between the 1920s and 1940s, Baghdad's population tripled—reaching more than half a million. During and as part of the DRB's development imperatives, in the early 1950s it began implementing plans for large-scale projects in the city. State-owned land was being transformed into neighborhoods and suburbs for rising numbers of civil servants and middle-class professionals. Electricity grids, clean water supply, waste collection, sanitation networks, and transportation were expanding thanks to increased infrastructure spending. Numerous modern bridges were erected to connect different points across the river, facilitating the movement of vehicles and people between the two sides of Baghdad carved by the course of the Tigris. Iraqi and international architects and artists were commissioned to contribute to the city's public planning by designing government buildings, public parks, sports stadiums, cultural centers, and public art.[24] The DRB invited internationally renowned architects, such as Le Corbusier, Walter Gropius, and Frank Lloyd Wright, to contribute to the construction of modern monuments in the city. Cinema houses boomed, showing the latest releases of Western, Indian, and Egyptian cinema. Restaurants, professional clubs, and nightlife spread across the city, offering to entertain the growing middle class.

In 1956, the British firms Minoprio & Spencely and P. W. Macfarlane presented to the board the first master plan for Baghdad. The plan outlined zoning principles and a system of roads and bridges. While work on these projects was underway, early in 1958 the board charged the Greek architect Constantinos Doxiadis from Doxiadis Associates with presenting a more expansive master plan for Baghdad, one that would accommodate the quickly growing nation's capital and address the problem of housing for the urban poor. Doxiadis and Associates had already been working on designing and executing a number of housing projects for Baghdad, Mosul, Kirkuk, and Musayyib. The board commissioned Doxiadis to design the capital's master plan because it wanted to be seen as choosing a "neutral" figure, thereby avoiding accusations of "imperial stigma."[25]

Doxiadis's work was centered on the notion of Dynapolis, the dynamic city—a neologism he used in his writings on city planning.[26] One objective of this model was to allow for the functional expansion of the city to incorporate unpredictable population growth. Doxiadis set the future limits of the capital's population growth at 3 million—a three-fold increase from 1958 population estimates. Neighborhood design included the zoning of communities. He believed that by developing "proper group-ings" among the different inhabitants, it would create "a healthy commu-nity spirit." An example of "proper grouping" meant "the insertion of middle-class housing between upper- and lower-income neighborhoods so as to minimize direct contact between opposite sides of the economic spectrum. Some residential sectors were even separated with 'green spaces' that acted as soft barriers among classes."[27]

This administrative ordering of social life fell short of dealing with the ongoing crisis of rural migration into the capital. While Doxiadis was drawing up his urban zoning of Baghdad's Dynapolis, informal set-tlements across the axis of the river were expanding in the capital. They became known as the *sarayif*—resembling the lodgings used in the south-ern marshland, from where many of the migrants hailed.[28] These mud-and-reed dwellings expanded to form close-knit clusters of homes, small passages, and markets. The peak of the migration came during the sum-mer, when river levels became low, hindering irrigation, and the summer's high temperatures favored the spread of sickness. Although some of the migrants hoped to return to the land, most ended up staying in the city.

The largest of these settlements was in the Karadat Maryam district on the western side of the river.[29] The migrants called their new homes, *al-'Asima* (the capital). Not withstanding the irony, the name was derived either from the shortening of 'Arasat al-'Asima (public land belonging to Baghdad municipality) or from the term for one of the first large settle-ments of the early migrants to the capital.[30] In official correspondences, al-'Asima came to be known as Khalf al-Saddah (behind the levee)— in reference to the government-owned wasteland behind the Nadhum Pasha dike on the Tigris. According to government estimates from the mid-1950s, al-'Asima housed close to 40,000 people.[31] Most hailed from Amarah, where they originally lived and worked on the vast agricultural lands straddling the Tigris and Euphrates, where the government had established the Dujaila settlements.

The settlements' proximity to the river was vital for the domestication of the livestock that the migrants brought to the capital. Maintaining the livestock was essential as a source of income. Herds of water buffalo were led daily to immerse in the Tigris, essential for their cooling down from the heat. It also encouraged the animals' milk productivity and reproduction. Men sought work as unskilled laborers in government, service, and in the industrial sectors then booming in the capital. Some worked as office boys, others as taxi drivers, builders, and wage laborers. Scores of men also enrolled in low-ranking positions in the police force and the army. Women brought in additional income by taking care of children, serving as domestic laborers, and marketing cow and water buffalo dairy products. For many of these women, this division of labor was a major setback; back on the land they were more central to agricultural work.

The presence of the *sarayif* and living conditions there acquired different valences in discourses about the city. The "ecology" of al-'Asima contrasted with the urbanization zeal that had befallen the capital, producing a complex moral economy of abjection. For Baghdadi urbanites, the presence of the *sarayif* at the heart of the city was an anticlimax in the city's modernization story. It reinforced the idea of the incommensurability of urban and rural societies. The inhabitants of the *sarayif* were resented as an inferior cast of *shroug* and *mi'dan*. The term *shroug* (sing. *shrougi*), or "easterners," designated those hailing from rural areas east of the Tigris; *mi'dan* (sing. *ma'idi*) indicated villagers who descended from Iraq's southern marshes.[32] The use of the term *shroug* also had a broader geographical genealogy. Both the *shroug* and *mi'dan* were traced back to descendants of historical migration from South Asia who had integrated with the tribes east of the Tigris and the southern marshes.[33] According to Ali al-Wardi, resentment toward the *shroug* and *mi'dan* was very strong, not only among the urban population but also among the other tribes of the western Euphrates, who saw them as untrustworthy and having an impure Bedouin lineage.[34] On a different note, the poor's social and economic conditions gave more traction to the Iraqi communist party, whose political program centered on social justice and the reform of the exploitative *'iqta'* system, and whose base was expanding among Iraq's dispossessed classes.[35]

Among development and public health experts, the burgeoning "rural slums" in the city were further fraught thanks to their "unhygienic" dwellings and "backward" cultural practices. Doris Phillips, an economist who wrote about al-'Asima during the 1950s, described the settlement as a "world in itself" with "ties with the city being through the labor market."[36] She contrasted it to the common configurations of "urban slums" generally:

> [Al-'Asima] has its own bazar, composed of tiny mud and reeds stalls, where lengthy bargaining takes place over foods rejected by downtown markets. It is more noticeably tribal in culture than are slums which are in closer contact with urban influence: most young girls are put in the black cape and headdress, to shield their charms from male eyes, several years before puberty; the cosmetic kohl is commonly seen around their eyes; and much of the dowry is spent on gold jewelry, as in the marshland from which many of them came.[37]

The lodgings of these "tribal slums" were further enmeshed in the pathological conditions of their adapted living space. Quoting a public health report by Critchley, Phillips explained:

> This area was the waste land to the East of the bund which surrounds Baghdad, and it was a desert site studded with pits of varying sizes, which have been produced by the excavation of mud and clay for building purposes. The area was also used by the Municipality as well as private individuals as a dumping ground for human and animal excreta, and rubbish. In addition the few surface water drains in the East of the city are pumped over the bund into this area, just after receiving the washings from the city abattoirs. The polluted and foul smelling liquid, which formed a sizable stream, wound its way through the conglomeration of mud buildings. . . . There were no sanitary arrangements in the houses or in the district, hence the inhabitants simply defecated indiscriminately, adding their small contributions to the already grossly polluted ground.[38]

In her words, Phillips further elaborates on the poor sanitary conditions and social anxieties produced by this amalgamation:

Conditions of sanitation are worse than their village of origin, by virtue of their greater numbers and density, but established urban people living near the al-'Asima are troubled more than are the Asima dwellers, who have had little experience with urban sanitary facilities. In most components of their real income, particularly diet, clothing, and household possessions, they are better off than they were before. They are aware of it: despite their many complaints, the overwhelming majority have no intention of returning to the farm. Their failure to make use of free social services is partly a result of fear and ignorance. Probably also it is a result of the established place in their standards held, for example, by meat, gold jewelry, and traditional types of household equipment—more than by literacy or good health, with which their experience is limited. Certain changes have occurred in their consumption patterns. The radio is a recent and politically important addition to the possessions of a small but significant proportion of Asima families. The men make use of some urban amenities, as for example the cinema, but their social life centers around the local coffee houses, as in the village. The life of the Asima women has changed relatively little, with exception of the few who have entered the labor market; however, it is very much easier than it was in their villages of origin, where they not only carried fuel and water and baked the bread but performed much of the agricultural labor as well.[39]

The fears about the abject conditions of the *sarayif* were heightened during the 1954 flood that hit the capital. The rising water levels from the melting snow in the mountains, augmented by the back flow from the newly constructed dams along the Tigris, inundated the city and different towns and agricultural lands along the river's path. The flood was considered one of the worst in the capital's modern history. The river water destroyed crops and threatened government buildings, markets, and residences close to the riverbank. The estimated loss from destroyed crops was put at 3 million pounds. The government declared a state of emergency. Both the military and the police were deployed to rescue those who were caught in the flood. State-sponsored radio aired songs and poems to mobilize the general population of the city to rise up to the occasion. Close to 250,000 people were evacuated from the low-lying areas in and around Baghdad. One of the flood's casualties was the *sarayif*, whose displaced residents took their livestock over the dike to camp in empty lots across the capital. Troubled by their dispersal through the capital, and the rising risk of disease brought by the flood, the government went so far as to force shanty residents to return to their original informal settlement once the waters had subsided. The migrants were reluctant to return to their dwellings near the river and "their squalid existence so easily observed for several months left a lasting impression after water receded and they were forcibly removed back."[40] Further contributing to the tensions about the future of this "urban–rural" cohabitation was the smallpox epidemic then afflicting the capital.

Instructed by the prime minister, the development board decided to raise its allocation for building public housing. The plan promised to build close to 30,000 housing units between 1956 and 1960 to accommodate the homeless migrants and those affected by the flood. These measures also came to address the rising political tensions following the 1956–1957 Suez crisis. Popular riots ensued, with protestors demanding that the government withdraw from the Baghdad pact, which guaranteed the country's alliance to the Western bloc during the Cold War.[41]

In 1957, the government sent wrecking teams "cutting swaths through al-'Asima for streets, and there was talk of drainage, electricity, plumbing, public baths and latrines, clinics, and schools."[42] These projects would never be realized. Instead, the foundation of a royal palace intended to house the eighteen-year-old king and his future bride was being erected in al-'Asima. Attempts to manage the social and medical threats posed by Baghdad's informal settlements were disrupted by political events, and the young king would not live to celebrate the inauguration of his new palace. On July 14, 1958, months before the inauguration, a group of young officers led a military coup that overthrew the monarchy. In a public spectacle, the young king was killed, and his body was disgraced along with those of members of his family and some prominent political figures. The migrants' future would be shaped by the post-1958 republican regime's social policies. The young King Faisal

II's unfinished palace was inaugurated as the "republican palace"; from here, successive Iraqi regimes would govern the country over the next decades. In 2003, the palace would be expanded and become part of the heavily guarded headquarters of the US occupation authority and the US embassy—known as the infamous "green zone."

"Revopolis"

The 1958 July revolution, led by 'Abdul-Kareem Qasim (1914–1963), ended close to thirty-eight years of British-backed monarchy in Iraq and defined the socialist path of the government. It declared the country to be a republic and instated a revolutionary council to manage government affairs. An army officer who came from a poor background, Qasim's promises of wide-reaching social change had wide popular support among the country's less-privileged classes. Qasim declared: "Social justice and higher standards of living for all." Determined to undermine Britain's political influence in Iraq, Qasim nationalized the territories owned by the Iraqi Petroleum Company and withdrew Iraq from the Baghdad pact. Qasim reinvigorated political ties with the Soviet Union and began negotiations to join the United Arab Republic (1958–1961), the short-lived union between Ba'thist Syria and Nasser's Egypt.

During Qasim's rule, Iraq witnessed very rapid state socialization with a focus on bringing the countryside under state protection. Qasim's most renowned legacy was his effort to address the conditions of landless farmers in the capital. Three months after the revolution, the Iraqi government passed the Agrarian Land Reform Law, which nationalized privately owned agricultural land and led to the dismantling of *'iqta'*.[43] The land reform was an attempt to curb the political and economic power of the landed classes. The reform, however, was not as radical as anticipated. "[The] land reform intended not to destroy the old landed classes as much as to neutralize them and possibly even lead them to become auxiliary allies within a reformed nation."[44] The Land Reform Law attempted a large-scale redistribution of land holdings to landless farmers. At the same time, it allowed for smaller private ownership of land by the remains of the landed classes. They were seen as an important asset to Iraq's emerging class structure and to the bourgeois stage of development.[45]

This transition to a semisocialist economy in rural Iraq was not a smooth one. Although land reform offered landless farmers the opportunity to own and reap a larger share of the crop, many farmers found themselves incapable of bearing the new responsibility. After years of oppression and exploitation by tribal landlords, who had assumed bureaucratic and technological control over the means of production, many farmers were unable to take charge of farming technologies, such as mechanized farming or sell their harvests directly on the market. In the two years following the revolution, southern Iraq witnessed other calamities that drastically affected agricultural productivity. Drought afflicted 1959 and 1960, but 1960 also witnessed an epidemic of equine fever that "destroyed thousands of horses, animals necessary not so much for transportation as for turning water wheels and, even more importantly, for plowing."[46] Many of the prerevolutionary development projects were also starting to fall apart. In a visit to Musayyib in 1964, Robert Fernea describes the state of disarray in one of the largest sites of prerevolutionary resettlement projects:

> [The visit] revealed long sections of canals and drains clogged with mud and water weeds, while government housing, built for the new settlers at considerable expense, stood largely empty. A few sections of this costly project land were under cultivation, but other areas were unfarmed and used for grazing flocks of goats and sheep. A number of tracts of land were completely bare and bright with salt crystals, indicating salinization of the soil—the curse of agriculture in much of Southern Iraq. The managerial machinery necessary to keep cultivator, land, and irrigation system in proper relationship had apparently been unable to cope with the complex problems presented by this agrarian innovation.[47]

Although a constellation of ecological and social forces contributed to the low productivity of land during the postrevolutionary years, more permanent options for the landless families were becoming available in the city. In Baghdad, the revolutionary council dismantled the DRB; its contracts with international companies and foreign experts were put on hold. The government rechanneled the projects to local Iraqi experts in government ministries, setting new priorities for the country's social reforms, with an eye to addressing the migrant populations and their informal settlements in Baghdad. The experts at the ministries revived the plans of Doxiadis's urban housing project in the peripheries of east Baghdad.

The original project was designed to cover twenty square kilometers of vacant land. It was marked to the west by a newly dug river canal that was intended to protect greater Baghdad from flooding. Doxiadis had designed the project as a gridiron—consisting of five to six districts, each with its own shopping centers, dispensaries, schools, mosques, and administrative buildings. Each district contained twenty-eight to thirty-two neighborhood blocks. In turn, each block was designed to furnish twenty-six to twenty-eight one-and-a-half-story housing units of 120 square meters. On each block Doxiadis had designed cultural spaces that he called "gossip corners," where the neighborhood communities would gather to socialize and exchange news.[48]

During the republican era, the new housing project became unofficially known as al-Thawra City (Revolution City). Plots of land were offered to low-income families and those who lived in informal settlements across the city. As soon as news of the project spread across Iraq, waves of migration to the capital spun out of control. More peasants claimed plots in the new state welfare project, joining family members and tribal kin. Pressure on the government mounted to distribute the land even prior to the completion of the service infrastructure. The government attempted to accommodate most of the applicants and invited people to submit architectural plans for their housing and business projects. People submitted rudimentary sketches drawn personally or by an *'ardhahalchi*—a literate entrepreneur who sits outside government offices filling out government paperwork for a fee.[49]

The state's attempts to remedy the problem of rural migration and improve the living conditions of the city's dispossessed farmers once again backfired. Many al-Thawra inhabitants kept their connections with their provinces through their tribal and family networks in the south. During the next decades, al-Thawra continued to receive rural migrants who had

abandoned their land and moved to the capital in search of better opportunities. Soon, the original six planned districts expanded to eighty, and
the unregulated construction of housing and shops challenged the project's
unfinished infrastructure. Open spaces turned into piles of waste and gar-
bage. Al-Thawra became Baghdad's largest urban ghetto.

The unfinished infrastructure and accumulated waste inside al-
Thawra continued to generate public health problems for the authorities
and defined discourses about the backwardness and uncleanliness of its
inhabitants. During the 1960s and 1970s, al-Thawra became a stronghold
of dissident political activities—especially those of the communist party.
In the 1980s, the city was renamed Saddam City, and political activists
there endured regular crackdowns by Ba'th Party paramilitaries and government security forces. One of the main contested aspects of the space
was the open sewage system that was left unfinished from the Qasim
era. The large septic tanks in each house collected excrement and water,
which drained, untreated, into the streets' open sewers.

Inspired by clandestine communist activities in Warsaw, dissidents
put documents and other literature in plastic bags and hid them inside
these septic tanks. Sometimes fugitives, too, immersed themselves within
to hide from government agents, who rarely looked inside the cesspits.
In the mid-1980s and during the Iran–Iraq war, the regime ordered the
completion of al-Thawra's closed sewerage system. Septic tanks were buried, and a new sewage system linked al-Thawra to that of the city. The
sanitation project, which dramatically improved the sewage collection
from the city, also marked the end of most clandestine communist activities in al-Thawra.[50]

Today, the forgotten archeology of al-'Asima stands for the deep
and complex dynamics of Iraqi statecraft—a product of miscalculated
development projects, social inequality, and the side-effects of state-
building policies. Nothing better captures these discontents than the
ominous concluding remarks of Phillips in her al-'Asima study:

> Town planning is frustrated by the migration, not only because it con-
> tributes an element of unplanned growth, but also because many authori-
> ties fear that furnishing amenities to the hut dwellers will accelerate the
> migration—as it may prove to do. Yet the health of the established urban

people is jeopardized by the ring of villages surrounding the city. Unsanitary practices have consequences in a community of 40,000 quite different from the consequences in an isolated village of a few hundred. The inability of the medical authorities to bring the recent smallpox epidemic rapidly under control emphasized to wealthy Iraqis the necessity of supplying sanitation and medical care to the urban slums, if for selfish reasons alone.[51]

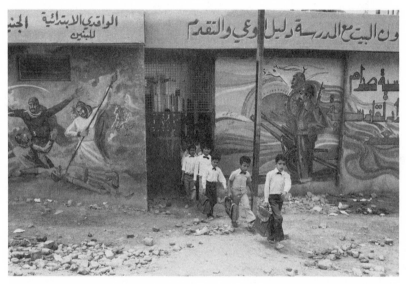

Elementary students leave their school in Baghdad, 1984. Scenes on the wall depict the
Iraq–Iran war.

6

Infants and Infantry

we are marching to war
like a lover who defends his beloved
this Iraqi, when he falls in love,
he perishes before a foe touches his beloved
we are marching to war,
so the nation remains safe for our generations
so childhood and play do not burn with our enemy's flames

1980s popular war song

ON THE EVE of the Iran–Iraq war, Salah Hashim, a bright young high school graduate from al-Thawra City in Baghdad, was finalizing his enrollment at Basra Medical College. His family had moved to Baghdad from Amarah and settled in al-Thawra during the reign of 'Abdul-Kareem Qasim. Inaugurated in 1967, Basra Medical College was Iraq's third national medical school. When the Iranian attack on the city began, Salah returned to Baghdad to stay with his family awaiting government notification to return to school. A couple of months later, classes resumed and Salah traveled back to Basra to begin his six-year training program.

During the eight-year conflict, Basra became a regular target of Iranian assaults. Located by Shatt al-Arab, Basra is only thirty kilometers away from the border. On several occasions the Iranian military attempted, unsuccessfully, to occupy the city with the intention of cutting off Iraq's only port city and its largest oil producer. Like other border cities in the country, Basra suffered heavily during the war. The city underwent many air raids and received regular mortar shellings from the Iranian side. During the bombings, the Iraqi government restricted movement out of Basra, due to the fear of a massive displacement from one of Iraq's largest cities—as was happening in other Iraqi towns and villages along the extensive border with Iran. Only those who could prove that they originally resided in other governorates could leave Basra. Military checkpoints on the main routes out of the city and in the main bus stations multiplied in order to check travelers' birth certificates. During attacks everyday life was disrupted. The city would adhere to blackout regulations, which usually restricted electricity usage for a week, sometimes longer. Shops and schools would close. Home windows and car headlights were painted blue to evade detection by Iranian warplanes. The medical facilities were the one place in the city running like a beehive.

The Basra Medical College's buildings and the hospital were frequently in the crossfire. At the college, classes ran daily from 8:00 a.m. to 4:00 p.m. The main basic science building is located in Tanouma on the eastern side of Shatt al-'Arab. During the conflict, the Republican Hospital—Basra's main public hospital—was hit few times by mortar rounds. During the shelling the college administration would move students to other buildings across the river. Basra's hospitals often received the overflow of injured soldiers from the nearby frontlines. On different occasions surgical wards of the city's main general hospital were evacuated to free up beds for the wounded. Operating rooms would cancel their elective surgery schedules to manage the hundreds of soldiers that poured in daily. Hospital staff, including medical students and faculty members, ran back and forth from the emergency rooms to the operating rooms to treat lacerations, fractures, and head injuries. Deep wound debridement and straightforward amputations were performed in the emergency room—in order to keep the operating rooms free for more complex surgeries. Doctors and specialists from across the country, especially from the capital, traveled on government assignment to frontline cities to perform more complicated surgeries. Senior surgeons signed up for a rotation in which they organized these assignments according to needs and during the intensification of battles. One leading Iraqi trauma specialist described the volume of his work during these days: "I would usually perform more than fifty operations in one day. These were only the facial and head injuries. We had a whole team of surgeons working together to deal with the different kinds and extents of wounds." Hospitals, such as the one in Basra, were sites of training and for the cultivation of knowledge and experience in clinical medicine and war triage. For doctors like Salah, there was a sense of pride and accomplishment, being able to be mentored by such teams. "We were trained by Iraq's best surgeons at the time," he recalled admiringly.

Iraqi doctors often remember the eight-year conflict with Iran with ambivalence. The war had brought loss and tragedies to every single Iraqi home. It was a period of repression and fear of the brutality of the ruling regime. Many doctors who served during the war relate horror stories of dealing with the immediacy of life and death on the battlefield. Iraqi doctors also remember that period as one of medical and public health achievements, of successes in cultivating knowledge and expertise in different medical specialties—a time of productive medical work. During the 1980s, international organizations also celebrated Iraq as a "success story" of a country reaching health and development milestones during wartime. Often-invoked achievements were the sharp reduction of infant and maternal mortality rates and the consolidation of rural primary care. One account expressed these achievements as follows:

> It is one of the paradoxes of Iraq's eight years of war with Iran that the conflict, which was the source of widespread suffering, also set the stage for substantial progress in child survival, especially among the "unreachable" rural population. In the midst of the war, Iraq was able to create conditions which cut the infant death rates by half: it fell from 89 to 40 deaths per 1000 live births between 1980 and 1989. This rapid decline in the rates of infant and child mortality due to neonatal tetanus, measles, polio, pertussis, diphtheria, and diarrheal dehydration reflected the increasing awareness and utilization of immunization, oral rehydration, and maternal and child health services.[1]

In this chapter I turn to this paradox of war and statecraft in Iraq. The eight-year Iran–Iraq war was among the longest interstate military conflicts of the twentieth century.[2] With accurate statistics absent, close to 1.5 million people were killed and injured on the two sides. The war represented a critical episode in Iraq's state-making history. From early on, the regime defined the war as one of survival against national and regional threats. It consolidated its repressive security apparatus and brutally eliminated its political opposition. The everyday realities of the war presented the state with much broader problems.[3] In response to battle-field losses resulting in death, the state focused on the expansion of its health-care services and cultivated the broader social significance of war-time "survival" and "productivity." The regime's mantra—"we fight with one hand, and we build with the other"—captured the interconnections between the war and social mobilization to respond to the "assault" on the physical and social body.

The aim of this chapter is not to celebrate the war as a form of affir-mative biopolitics, nor to undermine the great suffering that resulted from it. The experiences and memories of those who were killed, wounded, disabled, taken prisoner, or who went missing echo through Iraq's social and political fabric still today. I focus on the complex population politics and social dimension of that war that are often obscured or ignored in academic discourse on the conflict. As such, I interrogate the Iran–Iraq war as a terrain for the mobilization of different regimes of population-politics that shaped everyday life during the conflict. I focus on how Cold War–era state medicine and international health politics and organizations became implicated in the war and its consequences, and how, in turn, Iraq's wartime state managed to showcase a "productive" form of "body politic."

Revolutionizing State Medicine

To understand the Iran-Iraq war's impact on Iraq's medical infra-structure, it is necessary to note how the practice of state medicine trans-formed after the 1958 revolution and the way that enterprise was invoked to consolidate the health-care infrastructure during the war. The 1958 revolution introduced long-lasting and wide-reaching changes to the country's political structure and social and economic organization. It replaced the old oligarchy that had prospered under the monarchy and conditioned the emergence of new classes. Management of the coun-try's welfare institutions further consolidated the state's reach. After the revolution, development of the country's infrastructure was fast-tracked. The mobilization of medicine as an instrument of social and economic reform was central to this undertaking. In many ways, the revolution did not sever ties with the existing state medical enterprise. Instead, it rearticulated the limits of that system and promised to extend its reach.[4] This imperative was based on two main priorities: first, accelerating the expansion of health-care services and medical expertise; and second, reorienting the medical infrastructure to improving the health and social conditions of the rural poor.

The government criticized the monarchy's policies of favoring students from elite backgrounds and urged the popularization of medical study. After the revolution medical education became increasingly accessible to students from poorer and geographically remote backgrounds. As a first step in addressing the monarchy's shortcomings, the revolutionary council increased the state's health and education budgets. It increased student enrollment in existing schools and built more accessible ones in peripheral centers. During the first year of the revolution, the government changed the name of the Baghdad Royal College of Medicine to the Baghdad Medical College and boosted enrollment to 300 per year.[5] That same year, it inaugurated a new medical school in Mosul, which in its first year accepted approximately 123 students.[6] The government also opened a number of new nursing schools and promoted the enrollment of both men and women.

In the first couple of years, Iraq increased its number of hospital beds by 50 percent. Inspired by experiments in a number of communist states, the government introduced a new Ministry of Health program, *al-Siha al-Qarawiyyeh* or Village Health. This program received ample funding to expand the network of clinics and dispensaries, linking populations in cities, towns, and villages.[7] The government also used a system of "mobile clinics"—a small team of medics traveling in a specially equipped vehicle—to provide medical aid and vaccination, to peasants and tribes living in areas beyond the reach of small village dispensaries.

With its closer ties to the Eastern bloc, the government drew on medical expertise and resources from the Soviet medical enterprise. Before the first anniversary of the revolution, Iraqi and Soviet Ministries of Health signed a "Memorandum of Collaboration" to conduct a nationwide smallpox vaccination campaign in Iraq. In 1959, Iraq received a team of five Russian doctors, thirty nurses, and three translators to provide the vaccines and help carry out the campaign. The Russian team spent months traveling across Iraq to inoculate approximately 6.5 million people, 4 million of them in the countryside.[8] In addition, the team surveyed all primary schools and provided the "triple vaccine" (for diphtheria, pertussis, and tetanus) to first- and second-year elementary schoolchildren. The team also supplied small health centers and dispensaries across the country with the vaccine.[9]

With the popularization of medical studies came stricter rules regarding the organization of doctors' rural service. In 1961, the republican government issued *Qanoun al-Tadarruj al-Tibbi*, or the medical service law. The law aimed to enforce government service and to make registration for medical practice dependent on such service. If they failed to fulfill their obligations, physicians ran the risk of losing their license. Government service became more structured. Newly graduated doctors were distributed across the different governorate hospitals and required to rotate among major medical specialties—internal medicine, surgery, pediatrics, and obstetrics and gynecology. After two years of rotation, doctors were transferred to positions in one of the administrative subdivisions working in Village Health for one to two years. The new law translated into a more "proportional" distribution of doctors, especially in underserved governorates—some of which witnessed a 50 percent increase in the number of practicing doctors (see table).[10] Many physicians actually lived in the newly established health-care centers, which included a humble room for the local doctor with electricity and clean water. Although this did not fully solve the problem of doctors' reluctance, it reduced its incidence. Different forms of "favoritism" continued to be an important factor in determining the appointments of doctors.

Cultivating further scientific relations with the Eastern bloc's socialist experiments, the government opened new opportunities for studying medicine abroad in the Soviet Union, Romania, Poland, and East Germany. This created tensions with the generations of British-trained Iraqi doctors now in charge of setting standards for state medical-training programs. These doctors raised concerns about those returning from the Eastern bloc, who would have difficulty adapting to Iraq's tradition of "Western" medical standards and would be unable to communicate in

Iraqi Medical Doctors Distribution According to the Country's
Administrative Liwa's (1957–1962)

Liwa's	1957	1959	1962
Baghdad	592	714	758
Mosul	80	87	84
Basra	68	81	98
Karkuk	61	60	65
Diala	30	35	35
Karbala	28	46	61
Hilla	28	41	56
Diwaniya	28	32	37
Arbil	22	24	26
Nasriyeh	20	22	31
Amarah	19	22	24
Rumadi	17	31	47
Sulaimanyeh	16	23	36
Kut	15	27	27
TOTAL	1,024	1,245	1,385

English, the Iraqi medical community's primary language. Others worried about the increased number of students that local medical schools were absorbing. In a show of good faith, and in order to not disrupt Iraq's long tradition of medical training, the government continued to foster institutional ties with the British medical establishment. The Qasim government in fact raised the numbers of students sent to the United Kingdom to be trained in the different medicine specialties, among other professions. During that period more medical students were educated in the United Kingdom than in the Eastern bloc.[11]

Despite the popularity of Qasim's reforms among the general population at the time, political developments in the country soon put an end to his reign. In February 8, 1963, a military coup led by the Ba'th Party and other political factions stormed the Republican Palace, taking control over the government and killing Qasim after a mock military trial. Thousands of Iraqis were killed during the bloody coup. Over the next five years, a series of coups further destabilized the country, and in 1968, the Baʻth Party came to power.

Over the next decade, the Baʻth continued the social and medical reforms of the Qasim era. During this economically prosperous decade, the one-party state expanded social services—offering free public housing, extending national health care, and boosting the number of doctors and hospitals across the country. In 1972, the government nationalized Iraqi oil, and the Iraq Petroleum Company (IPC) was put in Iraqi hands. The government invested in doubling its refining capacities and laid a new pipeline across Turkey to the Mediterranean.[12] After the nationalization of its oil sector, Iraq benefited from a surge in revenue, thanks to soaring global oil prices. Development plans envisioned turning the country into a huge workshop to create employment opportunities. Massive literacy campaigns extended to rural and urban areas.

Having taken over the oil industry, the government led a campaign of administrative and bureaucratic reforms to shift the focus from "production" to "productivity." This meant focusing on improving rates of production among the employees and government institutions. These efforts were led by then vice president Saddam Hussein. They entailed restructuring ministerial organization to trim excessive and redundant procedures and lengthy bureaucratic processes. In that same vein, the state further embraced computing technologies to improve government efficiency. As early as the late 1960s, Iraq had already installed its first state computer systems to electronically manage electricity billing and other government services and industries.[13] One dimension of this reform was to foster a stronger "complaint line," encouraging citizens and government employees to pinpoint shortcomings in state bureaucracy.[14]

Oil nationalization and administrative reforms contributed to major leaps in economic and development indicators. Per capita income rose exponentially from $306 in the early 1970s to $3,734 in the late 1970s. The GDP reached an all-time high of $6 billion—fourteen times greater than that of the previous decade. Close to 63 percent of the GDP came from oil revenues. As one of Iraq's leading economists wrote: "Iraq had an economy where every indicator was showing high rates of growth by historical and contemporary standards—in relation to other countries.

Consumption, investment, exports, imports, infrastructure, and industry were all advancing at a fast pace."[15]

The influence of two decades of revolutionary reforms consolidated centralized state control and led to the expansion of welfare infrastructure. Despite the political turmoil during that period, Iraq's health-care and public health services continued to expand. By the start of the war with Iran, Iraq had tripled its number of registered doctors to 3,712. Hundreds of these physicians had taken specialist training in the United Kingdom. Furthermore, a network of health-care facilities had begun to show its "productive" role in bringing the countryside closer to state welfare.

Productivity in Wartime

In July 1979, Iraq's vice president, Saddam Hussein, led an internal coup in the ruling Ba'th Party leadership that forced Iraqi president Ahmad Hassan al-Bakr to step down. Hussein assumed control over the military and state security apparatus and went on to eliminate potential opposition both inside and outside the party. Thousands of people were exiled, jailed, or executed in attempt to take control and secure loyalty to his one-party rule of the country. The new president's rise to power coincided with mounting international fears that Iran's 1979 Islamic revolution might "spill over" to the Shi'a communities in Iraq and elsewhere in the region. After a few months of border skirmishes, on September 22, 1980, Baghdad ordered airstrikes on Iranian military airfields. The strikes aimed to paralyze Iran's airpower in preparation for a swift ground invasion. Iraqi troops advanced across the border to capture the Iranian port city of Mohammerah on Shatt al-Arab—about ten kilometers north of Abadan, the first locus of the 1923 cholera epidemic. Attempts at further territorial gains were futile. Casualties mounted to massive levels during the first weeks. As many as 5,000 Iraqi soldiers died, and close to 4,000 were injured in the battles of Khorramshahr—or the City of Blood, the Persian name of Mohammerah. Responding to the assault, the Iranian navy and air force launched a full-fledged attack on Iraqi military and civilian establishments. Iraqi military bases, oil facilities, dams, and oil terminals in the south of the country were some of the main targets.

The Iran–Iraq war was a critical turning point in the trajectory of state building and its focus on productivity. The regime originally envisaged a conflict that would end swiftly after impeding the Islamic Republic's military capabilities. The war was a bloody eight-year-long military stalemate. In the intervening years, Tehran refused to accept international efforts to end the conflict. The Iranian government depended on prolonging the war to drain Iraq's limited resources and force the regime to capitulate. During the first two years, Baghdad increased imports in an attempt to flood the market with consumer goods. At the same time, the state's military expenditure in the early years of the conflict reversed economic growth and threatened to undermine the previous decades' advances in development indicators. The foreign exchange reserve, which had amassed US $35 billion, was depleted rapidly.[16] The collapse in international crude oil prices in the 1980s expedited the decline in state revenue and the GDP. The Iranian military's targeting of Iraqi oil pipelines further disrupted oil exports. The longevity of the war and the rapid depletion of economic and human resources put the state under pressure. The flow of funds to Baghdad from the West and oil-rich Arab states of the Persian Gulf was not sufficient. In 1983, the Iraqi government declared it would confront inflation and other economic fallouts of the war with dramatic austerity measures. To support the national economy, most foreign imports that competed with locally produced commodities were banned. To prevent an exodus of populations, the government issued a travel ban, mainly on government employees and men of conscription age.

Confronting the Iranian army's superior numbers, the regime introduced strict conscription policies to the country's male population. Close to 1 million men were officially enlisted to serve in Iraq's two-tier armed forces: the regular and the Popular armies. Within five years of the start of the conflict, the regular army grew from 200,000 to 500,000, mainly through the broadening of the conscription age. On the other hand, "recruits" to the Ba'th-run paramilitary Popular Army reached close to 650,000, mainly through the recruitment of men above the official age of military service.[17] Most of the conscripts came from the socio-economic margins of the country—mainly Iraq's southern cities and towns. The military also depended on the underachieving school dropouts and students who were not able to enroll in universities or technical schools after taking the national baccalaureate exams. Education acquired greater social value because, above all, continued schooling in the overwhelmingly state-run education system guaranteed a delay in military service. This rise in the number of military conscripts paralleled the swelling number of doctors. During the war, the state expanded enrollment numbers nationwide and the number of doctors rose exponentially. By 1985, the numbers doubled, reaching 6,045 physicians.[18] In 1987, the state inaugurated four new medical schools in the governorates of Qadisiyyah, Najaf, Saladin, and Anbar. By 1989, Iraq could boast 8,808 registered physicians.[19] The military extended national service by one year for physicians. In addition to their rural service, doctors were required to work in military medical units and in support of military ambulatory care. Many doctors died serving on the frontline, and others were killed during the shelling of border cities.

During the early years of the war, government-sponsored scholarships for medical doctors to study abroad continued unabated. The Ba'th government favored doctors who were members of the party and gave them priority for such scholarships. After the start of the war, more doctors training in the West refused to return for fear of conscription. Many became dissidents, cutting their ties with Iraqi embassies to evade intimidation by government informants abroad.[20] In response to this rising tension with scholarship students, and under the umbrella of austerity, the Iraqi government terminated the decades-long foreign missions program. Physicians were strictly banned from travel, though a few were allowed to attend medical conferences abroad after acquiring myriad approvals from state internal security agencies.

The termination of the field specialization study-abroad program demoralized the younger generation of Iraqi doctors. Many had wished to use state scholarships to pursue medical training abroad. Meanwhile, senior Iraqi physicians were told to establish local alternatives. In 1986, the government approved the creation of the Iraqi Board for Medical Specialization. The board offered Iraqi doctors postgraduate training in different medical and surgical specialties and subspecialties. The board augmented the capacity of the regional postgraduate program, the Arab Board, which had started successfully a few years earlier. The government also inaugurated the subspecialties surgical hospital, al-Shaheed Adnan, in the Baghdad Medical City Complex. With a capacity in excess of 500 beds, the hospital became one of Iraq's largest and was equipped with up-to-date surgical technologies. It became the training ground for a new generation of Iraqi surgeons, vital for the treatment of wounded soldiers.

Iraq's medical infrastructure played an important role in managing the continuous flow of conscripts and ensuring their combat readiness. A committee at the Ministry of Health, composed of administrators, clinical specialists, and military doctors, determined fitness for service. It devised different kinds of medical exams and tests, deciding on each claim. There was a list of conditions, including both mental and physical disabilities, that excused a person from service. The reasons for exemption included a variety of conditions, such as bad eyesight, hypertension, diabetes, and medically defined psychiatric illnesses, to name a few. Men who claimed to be unfit for the war endured thorough medical examinations to decide on their lack of suitability for military service. For the rest, there were two categories: *salim musalah* (fit and armed) described the absence of medically identified physical or mental problems; and *salim ghair-musalah* (fit and unarmed), which was used for those who were considered fit for service but not for handling weaponry. Throughout the years the fitness threshold was lowered to qualify a broader population. Even those who were declared fit for unarmed service for such reasons as eyesight problems or amputation were drafted into a special military unit called *Sharhabil*, where they worked in various administrative jobs away from the frontlines.[21]

State population politics metabolized on multiple levels, going beyond the identification and management of "war population" and the mobilization of medical doctors. The Iraqi regime looked beyond its biomedical resources to respond to war losses and challenges to its economic productivity. Conscripting the male population into the military undermined the country's labor force. This had serious repercussions for the country's highly centralized governmental sector. With financial and human resources dwindling, the government defined new strategies of economic survival. To help cope with the manpower shortage, the state opened the door to Arab labor immigration. Priority was given to Egyptians, a large population that was dealing with the socio-economic dislocation caused by President Anwar al-Sadat's "liberalizing" policies.[22] Filling low-wage menial jobs in construction and agriculture, it is estimated that more than 1 million Egyptians worked in Iraq during the 1980s. This was probably the largest population of migrant labor working in any Arab state at the time.[23]

Because many men were mobilized to the frontlines, more women took on responsibilities as heads of household and active participants in the country's labor force. The war saw more Iraqi women enter social, economic, and public life, assuming more active, "productive," and "reproductive" roles in Iraq's wartime society.[24] Decades of progressive social policies that favored and supported female education paid off.[25] Increasing numbers of women were hired for low- and middle-ranking administrative and technical positions in Iraq's public sector. In a number of ministries, women employees constituted between 60 and 80 percent of the workforce.[26] Improving work conditions for women and providing an infrastructure for managing their family "duties" further facilitated women's incorporation into government jobs. Women's pay was increased and maternity leave was extended. At each government ministry, daycare services for working women with preschool-age children were provided.

The visible participation of women in the workforce contributed to international perceptions of Iraq as a progressive secular state. Its image appeared more "secular" than that of the Islamic Republic, which had legislated a "modest" public dress code for women. The Ba'th Party made use of this image to propagate the narratives of backwardness it ascribed to Iran, and it was critical to rallying support from the international community.

Women's role in the new war economy was not limited to their labor. The government also tapped women's personal resources. The Ba'th Party conducted donation campaigns across the country—known as *Hamlat al-Tabaru' Lil Majhoud al-Harbi* (Donation Campaign for the War Effort). Through coercion and cooptation, women lined up outside party headquarters to contribute money and gold jewelry. Although such policies stirred resentment toward the regime, it was seen as being balanced by a new social contract—defined by women's economic visibility and assumed independence. Women's precarious responsibilities toward the state were enmeshed in a strategy of national survival that depicted them as bearers and protectors of the new generations.

The Survival Experiments

Different geopolitical and international interests intersected in defining the scale and longevity of the Iran–Iraq conflict and contributed to the reengineering of state population politics during the war. The success of Iraq's wartime child survival campaign illustrates the interconnectedness of these interests. This community of interests was conditioned by Cold War politics and competing international and public health discourses and practices.

The start of the war in Iraq coincided with the development of two paradigms central to international health organization in the global south—namely primary health care (PHC) and the child survival revolution. In 1978, the World Health Organization (WHO) held a historic conference in the then Soviet city of Alma Ata. The conference brought together 134 countries and 67 international organizations and culminated in the Declaration of Alma Ata. Signed by all participating countries, the declaration gave international support to PHC—focused on low-cost, universal, and community-based preventative and curative health interventions. The declaration was considered a triumph for Eastern bloc states with universal health-care systems that depended on state patronage and public funding. The declaration attested that health was a "fundamental human right" and that governments should strive to attain the highest level of public health.[27] The declaration set out an ambitious global goal of "health for all by the year 2000."

Months after the Alma Ata conference, representatives from Western states met in the Rockefeller Foundation Bellagio in Switzerland to revisit the scope and ramifications of this global health agenda. The participants criticized the PHC framework as being too broad, utopian, and unrealistic. Instead, the meeting embraced what was then being championed as selective primary health care (SPHC)—a prioritization of health spending driven by market-based considerations.[28] SPHC advocated cost-effectiveness and economic feasibility—inspired by the neoliberal economic logic of the time. The SPHC approach recommended focusing on specific areas of population health and choosing effective treatments to address urgent health needs in economically overwhelmed developing states. SPHC was meant to curb the "overspending" of such states and their inability to repay their international debts. The proponents of selective primary health care adopted a population-based argument, giving priority to interventions that targeted the health of women and children in underdeveloped states. SPHC was an opportunity for the Western bloc to reclaim the international global health regime from the universalist agenda that appealed to socialist and communist states.

One of the main consequences of the adoption of the SPHC was the undermining the WHO and its global primary care agenda.[29] Western funding to the WHO was severely cut and channeled to UN organizations with specific population health initiatives—such as the United Nations Children's Fund (UNICEF). The latter's focus on the well-being of mothers and children seemed a good fit with the new structural readjustment approach of the SPHC. Over the next few years, the SPHC was scaled up and became integral to another international health framework, the child survival revolution.

In 1982, Jim Grant (1922–1995), then the incoming executive director of UNICEF, coined the term *child survival revolution* to address the staggering rates of death due to preventable diseases. With more than 15 million deaths globally—concentrated in the developing world—Grant emphasized the need for a new approach and a campaign that could at least halve this number. The rationale of the "revolution" was the mobilization of low-cost and simple interventions such as immunization and oral rehydration therapy (ORT) for the treatment of diarrheal diseases, especially among children. Immunization and ORT were deemed the "twin engines" of this ambitious child survival paradigm. One of the main aims of these interventions was going beyond saving lives and reducing infant mortality statistics. Child survival had to be integral to sustainable socio-economic infrastructure. The interventions promoted a lesser dependency on access to doctors, hospitals, and expensive medical technology. Instead, it encouraged social and community reorganization, such as training of traditional birth attendants (TBA), women-to-women education, and access to low-cost technologies, such as immunization and the administration of ORT.

In large measure, the child survival framework was effectively used as a critique of ongoing global conflicts and the conditions of children living in war. Grant saw children as a "zone of peace" and the global mobilization of his revolution as a way to mitigate the preventable deaths of infants and children in war. As former regional director of UNICEF, Richard Reid, argues:

> If a forceful demand for a period of child protection could be laid out persuasively, in comprehensive terms, to the antagonists in a conflict area, it might lead to more than calling a halt in the shooting to reach children. It could also be a dramatic demonstration of the potential force of the Convention on the Rights of the Child. And it could be an opening wedge for broader humanitarian interventions in war.[30]

UNICEF's focus on lowering infant mortality during the 1980s represented a convenient marriage between SPHC and the child survival revolution. It further spoke to a neo-Malthusian concern with global population control and family planning. Adopting this paradigm, UNICEF was on the verge of moving from small-scale projects, pilot studies, and field trials to supporting national campaigns in developing states that required a political commitment to mobilize resources and redefine social infrastructure.[31]

In Iraq, which was among the signatories to the Alma Ata declaration, primary health care had been implemented prior to the war, inspired by new attempts to restructure the public health-care system in the country with the help of the WHO. The start of the war was a blow to primary health care—especially with the waning of available state and WHO funding. Child survival acquired a stronger appeal with the state's focus on maintaining the productivity of the war economy. The focus on child survival was both strategic and tactical, tying together the lifelines of the family and the nation at war. At once, the cultivation of the future population guaranteed a population boom in the face of war losses. In a society that cherished children and extended families, these policies spoke to the cultural value of reproduction and resonated with the everyday uncertainties of sons and fathers killed in the war.

In many developing countries implementing family planning programs, child survival was tied to limiting family size as a means of population control.[32] The Iraqi case was somewhat different. The Iraqi government adopted pronatal policies, promoting higher rates of fertility and reproduction, and linked them to the strategy of war mobilization. The government adopted new policies regarding contraception. Although contraception was not actually illegal in the 1980s, it was definitely discouraged and was not readily available, as it had been before the war. Many incentives were given, such as the extension of maternity leave to one year—of which six months were paid. Baby food and articles were imported and subsidized.[33] In the workplace, the government established comprehensive daycare for employees and facilitated maternity leave and early retirement for women with three children and more. The government further offered loans, bonuses, and subsidies for young married couples. It regularly held public collective weddings, offering financial support for those who could not afford marriage expenses. With each child, married couples were entitled to an incremental monthly subsidy. The more children in a family, the larger the subsidy.

The role of both the WHO and UNICEF was critical during the war. As early as 1983, the government of Iraq began negotiations with the two agencies to reorganize its health-care system to integrate women and children's health, in compliance with the new international interest in primary care. The main goal was to focus on mobilizing state institutions and society to cut down on infant and child mortality through countrywide health promotion campaigns, outreach to rural areas, and active community participation. The new program emphasized the low-cost "stepping stone" to the full institutionalization of primary care.[34]

A critical agent in wartime mobilization was the Ba'th Party's women's organization, the General Federation of Iraqi Women (GFIW). Although it followed the mainstream policies of the party, the GFIW also functioned as a parallel institution to the male-dominated party hierarchy. The GFIW played a major role in pushing the child survival agenda and negotiating a broader role for women in terms of participation and equal rights, especially at the workplace.[35] The GFIW opened new offices across the country and established committees in all government ministries to facilitate women's employment. In 1983, the Iraqi government established a national Maternal and Child Health Council (MCHC). The council was chaired by the Ministry of Health and was constituted by representatives from the government sector and the GFIW. The council worked for the promotion and integration concepts and practices of maternal and child health in different activities and initiatives across the country. One of the main aims of its agenda was outreach to rural women and children. The new five-year plan defined the five pillars of the child survival program: maternal and child health (MCH), the immunization of children and pregnant women, the control of diarrheal diseases, daycare services, and social mobilization and participation. The program started workshops in different governorates, aimed at training health staff in primary care models with a focus on reproductive health services. From 1983 to 1986, the number of the MCH centers across the country quadrupled from 84 to 320.

Much of the work of the child survival campaign fell on the shoulders of the GFIW.[36] The GFIW devised a parallel plan to that of the MOH in its national conference and mobilized most of its budget to the campaign. The GFIW had 1.2 million members and depended heavily on volunteer work. The organization had 22 branches, 195 sub-branches, and 1,317 local units around the country. A decentralized structure of "community motivators" provided access to women from female party recruits from across the country. The GFIW further organized educational campaigns for women who were community leaders, primary school teachers, and field and factory workers.

The state mobilized other resources to advance the campaign. During the war, TV and radio broadcasts reached almost 90 percent of the country's landmass. Iraqi TV devoted close to three hours a week to the child survival program. The weekly TV program *Shams El 'Afia* (The Sun of Well-Being) addressed rural women's child and general health concerns via a dialogue between a mother and a community health motivator—at times with advice from a female physician. Daily newspapers and weekly magazines also addressed child survival activities on a regular basis. Health promotion posters decorated the different MCH centers regularly visited by women. One of the classic posters portrayed Sinbad and his friend Hassan, characters from a famous cartoon aired during the 1980s, hovering over a crowd of women and children on a flying carpet. A UNICEF ambulance with a human face gazed at the friendly looking nurse offering vaccines to a crowd of thrilled women carrying their babies in their arms. Stretching from side to side in Arabic, the poster read: "Accompany Sinbad in his happiness." At the top of the sheet, a health message read: "Our children are Iraq's wealth; protect this wealth with immunization."[37]

One of the main effects of this program was the wartime revival of the figure of the local midwife and her integration into the state healthcare framework. An earlier attempt to regulate local midwifery during the monarchy had been abandoned in the 1960s with the closure of the state-run national midwifery school. In the decades before the 1980s, the Iraqi state and medical community perceived the local midwife, or *daya*, as an antimodern figure, described her as backward and illiterate, and depicted her as contributing to unsanitary birth practices that had adverse effects on the health of mothers and children. Ministry of Health policies under republican and later Ba'thist rule emphasized the universalization of medically supervised hospital deliveries with outreach to remote rural communities. Under the influence of UNICEF's call to promote local midwives as a national and community resource for child survival, this policy was reversed in 1984. The new politically correct term for midwives was *al-Qabila al-Qanouniyyah* (licensed midwife), differentiating between those with state sanction and those without. The MCH program defined midwives as "a vital community-based resource for outreach programs, and began taking steps to promote the role of TBAs [traditional birth attendants] and overcome the resistance of the medical community."[38]

With wartime budget cuts and the move to low-cost primary care and child survival, the Ministry of Health took a critical decision to stop ongoing plans for the expansion of obstetrics and gynecology services to rural areas, infuriating medical doctors who resented the dependency on the backward tradition of midwifery. Instead of generalists and specialists, the decision was to train neighborhood and village midwives across the country and to integrate them in MCH centers and activities. In an effort to change negative attitudes toward nursing and midwifery in the country, the government reopened a midwifery school and encouraged young women to sign up. Wartime media and propaganda promoted nursing as an important patriotic profession.

The new training program for the local midwives went beyond "upgrading" their birthing practices. The long-term training program was "planned with the goal of re-introducing mandatory government licenses permitting TBAs to practice" and promoting other practices, such as the reporting of morbidity and mortality instances, and making the necessary referrals to local health centers.[39] Upon completion of the course, participating midwives received a one-year renewable government license. The program started with a month-long training course for 300 licensed midwives from Baghdad and its vicinity, with plans for "scaling up." Next, the program expanded to other urban centers and eventually to rural midwives.

Despite all the guarantees from the state and volunteers, the recruitment of rural midwives proved more difficult than anticipated. Many rural midwives had never held a government license before. Many were skeptical about their need for training and were reluctant to be away from home for an extended period of time. Some midwives feared government punishment for having practiced illegally and worried about their earnings being taxed by the state.[40] Responding to the midwives' demands, the course was shortened conveniently from one month to two weeks, and transportation was provided by local branches of the GFIW and the farmers' union. The midwives had to also accept regular supervision and monthly meetings with mobile health teams from the ministry.

The country's medical doctors resisted the idea of delegating birthing to midwives. A rift grew between those doctors who embraced this program as a critical public health intervention and those who saw it as a departure from earlier plans to expand curative care across the country. WHO and the Ministry of Health organized workshops for doctors at the national level to emphasize the role of primary care and preventive medicine over curative medical treatment. Doctors were given courses on maternal care and the importance of the child survival campaign. The ministry even attempted to rethink the medical curriculum by integrating PHC principles into it, a project that was not fully pursued.[41]

The wartime embrace of "child survival" transformed Iraq's healthcare institutions in multiple ways. With the new stress on community-based birthing and the role of women's organizations, the cultivation of child survival was displaced from a hospital-based practice to a community-based one. The program inspired more women doctors to specialize in maternal care and to integrate child survival paradigms into more traditional medical specialties, such as pediatrics, obstetrics, and gynecology. In contrast, more male doctors were lured to surgical specialties to address the load of wartime injuries and trauma.

The mobilization of the country's female population played a central role in the response to the war. It helped move the state to formulate a more nuanced agenda concerning productivity (and reproductivity). Child survival practices were articulated in the context of broader transformations in the logic of global health regimes and international health policies. It aimed to expand the country's fertility rates and help secure the survival of a new generation of Iraqis. Many international organizations deemed "child survival in wartime" an innovative program that showed the Iraqi government's "political will and commitment" to improving the "well-being of mothers and children."[42] The focus on children had a dual political effect. It guaranteed Iraq's international and political commitment to development and state making. At the same time, the focus on infant and child mortality fostered policies to normalize a wartime politics of survival and productivity. The expansion of state medicine and its dependence on alternative means of outreach further guaranteed the resilience of the country's challenged infrastructure. It also revealed the state's dependency on its different human resources at times of crisis.

Cautious Optimism

On August 8, 1988, Iran and Iraq signed a ceasefire agreement. In Baghdad, the news came as a surprise. Millions of Iraqis went out to the streets in a spontaneous celebration of the end of a brutal eight-year conflict. Parades of honking cars moved through the streets carrying the

Iraqi flag. People marched, clapping and chanting. Others stood outside their homes watching and throwing water from buckets and hoses as a sign of celebration. Celebratory gunshots could be heard across the city. The government declared the whole week a public holiday. The celebrations continued for weeks.

There was a sigh of relief and a sense of cautious optimism. At the level of government institutions, there were plans to revive prewar projects that had been frozen. Still, the state's finances were severely drained. Iraq emerged from the war with huge debts to Western and Gulf Arab states. There were promising prospects of import credits and loans from Washington, DC. Riyadh was willing to shoulder a big chunk of the loans from other Arab states. There was an emerging space for imagining a postwar society. Iraq's military industry had grown, and there were rumors of translating this knowledge and know-how for the sake of civilian projects. The Ministry of Oil began negotiating with the government about reactivating the Foreign Mission Program to cultivate a new generation of Iraqi experts in the United Kingdom.

On August 1, 1990, Iraqis awoke to the sound of war songs blasting from the state radio and TV. Many of the Iran–Iraq war songs were being re-aired. This time, it was a different kind of war. Overnight the elite Republican Guard stormed into neighboring Kuwait and occupied the whole country in a matter of hours. Many Iraqi generals did not even know there had been plans for such an invasion. In January 1991, the US-led coalition launched Operation Desert Storm, whose official aim was to quash Iraq's occupation of Kuwait. In the main, coalition forces devoted their energies to the strategic destruction of Iraq's physical infrastructure. Aerial bombardment and cruise missiles hammered Iraqi cities for forty days, dropping more than 90,000 tons of bombs. In Baghdad, bridges linking the two banks of the Tigris River were demolished, power stations were destroyed, and water sanitation systems across the country were ruined. Decades of infrastructure work had been undone. For months, Iraqis living in the capital had no electricity, no clean water, and no telephone lines. A popular rebellion in the south of the country further undermined regime control and provoked a brutal response that led to the death of thousands and the flight of many more.

The 1990–1991 Gulf War and its aftermath would define a new era in Iraq's state-building project. For the next twelve years, the economic sanctions crippled the state's capacity to restore the country's infrastructure. In contrast to the achievements in public health made during the Iran–Iraq war, the sanctions induced one of the worst and most alarming rises in infant mortality rates witnessed by any country in modern history.[43] The Gulf War the and subsequent sanctions regime triggered an exodus of thousands of Iraqi physicians and undermined Iraq's decades of institution building.

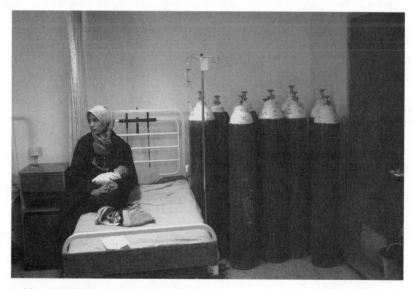

Saddam Children's Hospital, Baghdad, Iraq, 2002.
Photograph by Thomas Dworzak/Magnum Photos

7

Empire of Patronage

> The greatest cruelties of our century have been the imper-
> sonal cruelties of remote decision, of system and routine,
> especially when they could be justified as regrettable opera-
> tional necessity.
>
> Eric Hobsbawm, *The Age of Extremes: 1914–1991*[1]

THE DISMEMBERMENT of state infrastructure and the mass
exodus of Iraq's doctors under decades of US-led intervention has been
one of the central tragedies of Iraq's health-care system. This degradation
signified the loss of a critical mass of state doctors and undermined
decades-old modes of socialization and medical professionalization.
Leaving a "broken down" health-care system, Iraqi doctors sought to
find refuge in a "functioning" system that offered them the potential
of the universality of medical knowledge, up-to-date technology,
and opportunities to specialize in a branch of medicine they desired.
Decades of British institutional patronage made the United Kingdom
the obvious destination for many. Physicians' flight to Britain and their
integration into the National Health Service (NHS) is not merely a story
of "brain drain." The movement of Iraqi doctors to the erstwhile imperial
metropole speaks to the transnational genealogy of the Iraqi state. It is
one that continues to reverberate through the story of Iraqi medicine and
its entanglement in the practices and histories of empire.

In this final chapter, the ethnographic gaze is "displaced" to Britain, to explore the consequences of decades of war on the dismantling of
Iraq's health-care system through the flight of its doctors. These physicians' journeys demonstrate how personal, social, and professional factors
intertwined in the pursuit of asylum and labor outside Iraq. Doctors
risked dangerous journeys, paying off smugglers and human traffickers

in search of asylum in the United Kingdom. Once within Britain, Iraqi doctors sought to denounce their Iraqi papers, to acquire British nationality, and to settle and live in the United Kingdom. They were lured by the promise of a better life and career, in what many recognized as the extension of their professional world of medical training in Iraq. The experiences of Iraqi doctors in the United Kingdom attest to persisting legacies of the British Empire's scientific and patronage projects in its colonies, legacies that continue to shape the postcolonial medical-scientific infrastructure in Britain itself.

From Cradle to Grave

In 2005, I arrived in London to conduct research with Iraqi doctors in the United Kingdom. With the help of senior local physicians, I attempted to secure access to an NHS hospital in London. I planned to shadow different generations of Iraqis working in British hospitals to explore how they were faring, to interrogate their motivations and the possibility of their return to Iraq after 2003. In my request letters to hospitals, I elaborated on my research project and explained that I was an anthropologist who happened to be a trained medical doctor in Iraq. I explained that I did not have any intention of pursuing a career in the United Kingdom as a physician, and that I was ready to share all my findings with the hospital administration. My requests were systematically rejected. They explained that there were no available internships to offer me, that clinical shadowing positions were very competitive and exclusive to the few doctors who intern in British hospitals. For these hospitals, my Iraqi "nationality" and the fact that I was a trained medical doctor probably raised suspicions. At the time, the NHS was going through a major overhaul to limit the hiring of foreign doctors.[2] There were thousands of non-British doctors competing for these unpaid positions.

A few months after my arrival, the British government issued a new immigration law making it more difficult for non-European doctors to work or train in the NHS. The new rule marked a turning point in their organization, which undermined a decades-old custom of employing foreign doctors from Britain's former colonies. This was not the first time that the NHS cultivated "racial" tensions with overseas doctors. Since its inauguration in 1948—one year after Britain's withdrawal from

India—the NHS had depended heavily on a migrant labor force from the Indian subcontinent to fill the United Kingdom's health-care shortfall.[3] The anti-immigrant sentiments migrant doctors have faced tend to question the standard of medical training in their home countries, despite the fact that most had graduated from British-recognized medical schools. Until the mid-1970s, overseas doctors from such schools automatically registered with the General Medical Council (GMC)—Britain's main medical licensing body.[4] Since the late 1970s, recognition of these medical schools has been dropped, and overseas doctors have been required to undergo a range of written, oral, and clinical exams in order to be allowed to practice in Britain.

Overseas doctors were treated as second-rate physicians, whose skills and training were seen as inferior to those of British-educated practitioners. Over the course of its history, overseas doctors were given "marginal" jobs in the NHS. They were also often pushed away from "prime" postgraduate positions and had to occupy lower-paid jobs in remote or underprivileged areas—filling posts that the British doctor did not want. In parts of Britain, overseas recruits filled more than two-thirds of positions. The promotion of migrant doctors to a higher grade took longer than that of their white counterparts. To upgrade, immigrant physicians had to apply for more posts or change their career trajectories.[5] Following this, they were allowed to compete for only particular specializations—such as geriatrics, anesthesia, emergency medicine, and psychiatry—better known among the doctors as the "Cinderella specialties."[6] British-trained doctors sat at the top of the social and professional pyramid, while overseas doctors functioned as gatekeepers and second-class practitioners, whose presence was necessary to ameliorate the shortcomings of the NHS—Britain's largest welfare institution.

If the 1970s was a period of managing the qualifications of overseas doctors in Britain, then the 1980s represented a turning point in this relationship. The neoliberal reforms of Britain's Thatcher regime brought critical transformations to the NHS that echoed in its relationship with overseas doctors.[7] The reforms eventually led to the introduction of new decentralized administrative bodies, each of which functions as an independent self-governing trust.[8] These entities would compete for services in the internal market of the NHS.[9] A new managerial structure focusing on efficiency and productivity was introduced in the hospitals, which took decision-making power from doctors and placed it in the hands of newly appointed managerial boards. Hiring and firing was no longer a decision monopolized by doctors. It entailed a whole new bureaucratic process that also introduced uncharted NHS subspecialties and career tracks that had not existed before. With the shortage of such medical specialties, these positions opened up to overseas doctors. Despite the need to fill these positions, the government was reluctant to expand the number of registered overseas doctors.[10] Young immigrant doctors were still shunned from the "good specialties" and were generally accepted only in less-attractive postgraduate positions. Since then, the NHS has gone through one organizational crisis after another brought about by the competing logics of political and economic reforms. Such crises were often projected on Britain's overseas labor force. The 2006 rule and the disavowal of overseas doctors was only one episode in this history.[11]

On April 21, 2006, the new rule provoked hundreds of South Asian doctors to protest in front of the Department of Health in Whitehall. Many felt that the NHS had betrayed them.[12] Like their predecessors, these physicians had invested time and finances to come to the United Kingdom and work in its hospitals. The rule would leave close to 20,000 of them jobless.[13] The British government explained that the new rule was to align British labor laws with those of the European Union.[14] As a result, British hospitals were encouraged to hire EU doctors. The British government also declared that it was protecting these posts for UK doctors as supply outstripped demand.[15]

Not one Iraqi doctor attended these demonstrations, though the law directly affected their training opportunities. In fact, most doctors I spoke with were disinterested in antigovernment protests. For Iraqi physicians, the largest population of asylum doctors in the United Kingdom at the time,[16] their relationship with Britain had other dimensions. Many were on the track to becoming British citizens or had already done so.

Career Asylum

Many of the Iraqi doctors who arrived in the United Kingdom in the 1990s and the early 2000s settled after acquiring political asylum. Those doctors have taken many risks to find security in the West—good career opportunities and a better future for their kids. None of these immigrants left home under the illusion that things were going to be easy. On the contrary, they knew that the path to "making it" in Britain was a very difficult one. They also knew that the Iraqi doctor was appreciated in Britain, thanks to a history of institutional exchange and medical connections. They knew that scores of top-notch Iraqi consultants had been working in the United Kingdom for decades. Many had reached high positions in their careers. They strongly believed that their medical knowledge and rigorous training would allow them to compete with British and other migrant doctors. Many had studied medicine in English and spoke the language well enough in everyday interactions, which would make integration smoother. For many of these Iraqi doctors, such expectations were shaken by the realities of the world they had imagined. This was not necessarily a new cultural space to which they needed to acclimatize. Iraqi doctors recognized their entanglements in the structural impasses of the health-care system in which they hoped to work, as well as the broader regimes of power that produced their predicament.

The centrality of asylum policies and practices in shaping Iraqi doctors' path to the British labor market is illustrated in the migration story of an Iraqi physician named 'Ammar. I met 'Ammar a few months after my arrival in the United Kingdom at Sarchanar Restaurant, one of the handful of Iraqi diners in Northeast London. After finishing our greasy kebab, 'Ammar suggested that we head to the *gahwa* (coffee shop) to digest our food with some Iraqi cardamom tea. We also planned to watch a World Cup football game there. I had not seen 'Ammar in close to nine years. We had gone to high school together and trained at Baghdad Medical College during the 1990s. Only a handful of our colleagues remained in Iraq. A few had settled in Jordan. The rest were scattered across Europe and the United Kingdom, settling in and figuring out their careers.

We drove for a few blocks, stopping by one of the coffee shops frequented by Iraqis. The smell of apple tobacco smoke from the *narguilas* welcomed us as we stepped in. The place was just beginning to fill up in anticipation of the game. Customers were slowly congregating in front of the large plasma TV. Some had already fallen into discussions of the 2006 World Cup contest. In the far corner, a few customers sat at cheap plastic tables, slamming their checkers on backgammon boards, hurrying to finish their set before the start of the match. We took an empty table beneath a kitschy old poster advertising tourism to Iraq's Kurdish north. The poster was reminiscent of the Iraqi Ministry of Tourism posters that usually hung in the offices of Iraqi Airlines and offices of travel agents back in the 1980s. 'Ammar explained that the owner of the place was an Iraqi Kurd who had lived in Kuwait before the Iraqi invasion of 1990. He was kicked out of Kuwait after the Gulf War and joined other Iraqi Kurds in refugee camps in the south of Turkey.[17] Many of these refugees were eventually resettled in Britain. Other Iraqi refugees from the south, many involved in the failed popular uprising of 1991, were resettled from refugee camps in Saudi Arabia.[18] The rest of the asylum-seekers had claimed their status after entering the United Kingdom illegally. 'Ammar was among the latter.

Football was one of the main bonding and entertainment activities for Iraqis in the United Kingdom. When the game started, the mood in the *gahwa* changed to one of elation. We turned our chairs to face the TV. The French and South Korean teams faced each other in the play-offs. A football fanatic as long as I have known him, 'Ammar was very excited. He watched the English leagues regularly and knew all the players' names. I watched 'Ammar get into animated conversations with the other customers. They spoke of the different teams and star players and their tactics. The match went on with commentary from the customers.

The French team was mostly constituted of players of West and North African backgrounds. As one of the players missed a chance to score, 'Ammar stood up and waved at the TV, sarcastically announcing, "He is probably *mshagig*! The French will renounce his citizenship papers and smack him back to his home country." I did not understand what *mshagig* meant in this context. The Arabic adjective *mshagig* means "someone who tears up something." I turned to 'Ammar and asked him what he meant. "You have not lived in the United Kingdom for that long," he laughed, explaining that the player had obviously torn up his passport and was given "refugee status" to play with the French national team. It was a frequently used adjective among Iraqi migrants, describing how one tore up one's passport upon arrival before claiming refugee status. 'Ammar's comical remark was more than an analogy for asylum. It resonated with the predicament of many Iraqi doctors and the "illegal" journeys they'd taken to the United Kingdom and Europe. The doctor's escape from Iraq began with a counterfeit passport. In an attempt to curb their exodus, the Iraqi government had instituted a long-standing travel ban on doctors. Furthermore, the government and their universities withheld doctors' graduation certificates and grades. Doctors needed to obtain clearance and permits from the Ministry of Health, the Internal Security Forces, the Directorate of Conscription, and in some cases the Office of the President. Still, in 1990s Iraq, everything was possible for the right sum. The deterioration of everyday life under the sanctions regime and the inflation of the Iraqi dinar had made bribes a common income supplement for poorly paid government employees. A middle-ranking government employee received between $2 and $4 per month, which barely covered transportation costs to and from work. In certain cases higher-ranking government managers would collect such bribes and redistribute them among their directorate's employees to guarantee a fair and equal distribution of wealth. One thing was certain: the harsher the regulations against travel became, the more doctors were leaving illegally.

In 1998, 'Ammar left Iraq with a forged Iraqi passport that described his profession as businessman. He purchased his passport from *Soug Mraidi* in al-Thawra City—better known locally as *soug al-haramiyyah*, or the "thieves market," the hub for expertise in forgery of government documents and stamps. He then paid one of the handful of smugglers well-versed in trafficking medical doctors. They had a network of military and security personnel manning passport control desks at the Iraqi border. Arriving in Amman after a fourteen-hour-long road trip, 'Ammar had no intention of staying for more than a week. Jobs in Amman for Iraqi doctors were becoming limited, and Jordanian hospitals were exploiting the Iraqis' desperation by offering them low pay and minimal job security. For escaping doctors, the need to continue working as physicians was imperative. It allowed them to stay in touch with medical practice and filled possible gaps in their résumés when it came to applying for future posts. 'Ammar was unable to follow the costly path to asylum in the West immediately. A young middle-class doctor, he knew the expenses would be a heavy burden on his family in Iraq.

'Ammar's next destination was Yemen, where Iraqis were able to travel with no visa and where the Iraqi doctors had an excellent reputation. Yemen had opened its doors to Iraqi doctors in order to fill the vacuum of its own under-resourced health-care system. His plan was to save some money to cover part of the cost of the asylum journey to Europe. The rest of the money he would try to get from his family. 'Ammar spent nine months in Yemen working in a small health center on the outskirts of the capital, Sanaa. After a few months, he realized that he was saving very little money. "I was barely learning anything new in this ill-equipped clinic," he explained. Along with two other Iraqi doctors living in Sanaa, he decided to return to Amman to find other means to be smuggled to Europe.

With his Iraqi passport, 'Ammar struggled with limited travel options. During the 1990s, there were only a few Middle Eastern countries that allowed the entry of Iraqi citizens. With the strict regulation of the economic embargo on Iraq, regional governments systematically denied visas to Iraqis. Western countries also denied Iraqi visa requests— for fear of encouraging the influx of nonregulated asylum-seekers. One of the few alternatives available was an efficient Amman-based network of human traffickers that specialized in moving Iraqis into Europe. 'Ammar made contact with one of the facilitators, who promised to get him into the United Kingdom for $10,000. 'Ammar explained that the fact that the facilitator was a white Australian, assisted by an Englishman, gave him greater confidence about the "guarantee" of the journey. He had heard horrifying stories from other colleagues who had been forced to swim, walk for days, endure police abuse, or were abandoned in the middle of nowhere.

Needing financial help for his journey, 'Ammar contacted his family and explained his situation. The family had sold his car and kept the money aside for him. Official money transfers to and from Iraq, especially of such a large amount, were under scrutiny by the regime and the sanctions system. Instead, he received the amount through a family acquaintance living in Jordan. He paid half of the amount to the facilitator as a first installment. The rest of the money he promised to pay after his safe arrival in Thailand, where he would receive a counterfeit French passport to allow him to travel to the United Kingdom.[19] 'Ammar arrived safely in Bangkok. There, the facilitator took away his Iraqi passport and handed him a French passport and booked him on a flight to Beijing, where he would board a plane to London's Heathrow airport. Security at Beijing airport for flights to Europe is usually heightened. British customs officers usually board Heathrow-bound planes to check travel documents and deter illegal migration. 'Ammar's first attempt failed, and he was lucky that the officers did not detain him. On his second attempt, he sat at the back of the plane. British immigration officials checked more than two-thirds of the plane's occupants, and approximately forty passengers had been forced to disembark on suspicion of forged documents. At some point, the Chinese flight crew complained about the delays, and the British, perhaps satisfied with the size of their catch, left without checking the rest of the passengers.

Upon arrival at Heathrow, 'Ammar's instructions were very clear. He hid in one of the public toilets on the way to the passport control line. He needed to conceal any evidence that might betray his point of origin or how he came to London. He'd brought very good scissors to dispose of his fake French passport and, having reduced it to tiny pieces, flushed it down the toilet—except for the piece that had his photo, which he swallowed. When a few hours elapsed, Ammar left the restroom and surrendered himself to immigration authorities. He explained to the interrogation officer that he was a medical doctor who had escaped Iraq because of political persecution and that he wanted to pursue his career in Britain. 'Ammar said the officers were very polite with him despite his evasive answers. "They asked me about the airlines that I came on. I told them I didn't know. They asked me about the color of the airplane, I answered, white. They inquired about the flight attendants' uniform, I said white and blue. They knew that I would not tell them anything. They listened to my answers with a sense of sarcasm. They knew what was going on. They let me go. There was another Iraqi family, a woman with her child, waiting to be interrogated." The customs authorities asked 'Ammar to report the next day for a prolonged interview at the UK

Home Office, where he would file his asylum papers. 'Ammar stayed with a friend in London and went to the Home Office the next day. After going through another round of interrogation, the following interaction occurred: "They asked me where I wanted to live, I said, London. They explained that there was no way they would settle me in London. They suggested relocating me to Newcastle. They told me that there was a good medical school there!"

The overwhelming number of Iraqi asylum cases in Britain during the 1990s benefited from the many loopholes in the system. Asylum-seekers had to convince the immigration officers that they had pressing reasons to be granted asylum. After the 1991 Gulf War, human rights organizations often reported on the Iraqi regime's abuses against its ethnic and religious groups. This narrow, communitarian framing of the humanitarian situation in Iraq was appropriated by many asylum-seekers. Several of the doctors I spoke with explained that they were specifically asked if they belonged to one of Iraq's main "oppressed majorities or minorities." Some doctors felt very uncomfortable having to disclose their backgrounds. Others saw this as an opportunity to strengthen their asylum applications. They emphasized their affiliation with one group or the other. One colleague told me that his aunt, who came from a Sunni background, claimed to be Shi'a, just to make her case more appealing. During the 1990s, Egyptian, Lebanese, and Palestinian asylum-seekers posed as Iraqis in hopes of strengthening their cases. In an effort to curb such practices, asylum-seekers were often asked about specific neighborhoods in their cities to confirm their Iraqi origins. In many of these cases, the outcome of the asylum application process depended a lot on chance and on how much case officers were convinced by the applicant's story and performance.

Many Iraqi doctors like 'Ammar have taken similar journeys into Britain. The flight of Iraq's doctors during the 1990s was shaped by many variables. Doctors moved among different health-care systems of neighborning countries. Due to their precarious Iraqi documentation, they accepted low-paying positions in under-resourced health-care systems. Many felt that they were putting their lives on hold in order to find the right moment to relocate to the West. Doctors improvised and paid their way into the United Kingdom via human traffickers. The determination of Iraqi doctors to reach the United Kingdom came with hopes for better work opportunities and career prospects than those in Iraq or its neighboring countries.

Plab and Kebab

Once in the United Kingdom, there were many other hurdles to endure—namely acquiring registration and licensing to practice medicine, with the goal of finding a job in the highly competitive NHS system. 'Ammar was somewhat lucky on that front. He was resettled in a small apartment in Newcastle and given a weekly stipend. It took him about two years to finish the licensure and registration. After that, he landed a position in the NHS, working up the career ladder to become an anesthesiologist—one of the few available specialties for an overseas doctor at the time.

It is important to contextualize the history and the politics that shaped medical licensing practices for overseas doctors in the United Kingdom. As mentioned earlier, many of the doctors coming from Britain's former colonies were immediately registered with no required tests. The introduction of licensing for overseas doctors in Britain dates to the period of racial tensions during the mid-twentieth century. The British government's aim had been to regulate the flow of immigrants from the South Asian subcontinent. In 1965, the British Parliament introduced the first anti-discrimination bill, the Race Relations Act. In the face of strong resistance, the act had been promulgated to combat what was deemed the "colour bar"—customary practices of racial discrimination banning "non-whites" from using public spaces and resorts.[20] The act prompted anti-immigration riots, most memorably after British politician Enoch Powell made his infamous 1968 anti-immigration speech—better known as "Rivers of Blood." In his speech, Powell, who as a Minister of Health a few years earlier had called for recruiting doctors from India and Pakistan, warned against allowing the flow of migrants from the Commonwealth. The speech was followed by strikes, particularly in London's docklands, motivated more by support than opposition from the public.[21]

In the midst of this anti-immigration sentiment, voices emerged in the British media and among physicians questioning overseas doctors' standard of training. British doctors criticized what they saw as the "cultural incompetence" and the "substandard" levels of medical and communication skills among the overseas doctors.[22] In 1972, following Pakistan's withdrawal from the Commonwealth, the General Medical Council (GMC) withdrew automatic recognition from Pakistani medical graduates. That same year, the GMC withdrew recognition from Sri Lankan medical schools. At approximately the same time, the British government initiated a revision of its policies toward accreditations and its dependency on overseas staff. The government commissioned a committee, headed by physicist Alexander Merrison, to review the country's health system. Published in 1975, the Merrison Report dedicated a whole chapter to the issue of overseas doctors. It identified their presence as part of the larger "problem of external labor" in Britain:

> We believe that the inescapable conclusion to be drawn from evidence we have received is that there are substantial numbers of overseas doctors whose skill and the care they offer to patients fall below that generally acceptable in this country, and it is at least possible that there are some who should not have been registered.[23]

Criticism was voiced in professional medical journals about the controversial and far-reaching measures of the report.[24] The criticism came mainly from South Asian doctors on the grounds that not a single member of the report committee came from a minority ethnic group and that none of the committee members had either knowledge or experience of the "cultures and backgrounds" of overseas doctors or personal experience working with them in Britain or abroad.[25] Furthermore, none of the emerging overseas doctors' associations were consulted in gathering information or in the report's conclusion. Rather, "evidence" was generated from British members of the Royal College in Britain, whose membership was well known for their attitudes against immigrants in general. The report also fell short of recognizing Britain's changing demographics, with rising numbers of migrants from former colonies.

The government rushed to implement the Merrison Report's recommendations. This entailed a stricter stance on overseas doctors and what was seen as a belligerent dismissal of training in their home institutions. Prior to the report, the GMC recognized eighty-six overseas medical schools, fifty-five of which were in India. After the release of the Merrison Report, the GMC announced that recognition would be withdrawn from all Indian medical colleges.[26] That same year, the GMC set up the Temporary Registration and Assessment Board (TRAB) to test the medical and linguistic abilities of overseas doctors intending to work in Britain. The TRAB worked as a bottleneck through which the GMC controlled the employment of migrants in the NHS. In 1978, the GMC introduced a more comprehensive test to replace the old TRAB, named the Professional Linguistic Assessment Board (PLAB), which continues, to this date, to be the main licensure exam for migrant doctors in the United Kingdom.

The PLAB is designed to assess the knowledge and practice of doctors and their ability to work "safely in British hospitals."[27] It also tested overseas doctors' oral and written English skills. With some exceptions, the PLAB is required from almost all overseas physicians planning to work in Britain. It takes a minimum of one to two years to complete. Approximately half of the candidates who take the exam pass the test on the first trial. Many take the exam more than once. The PLAB consists of two parts: one entails a three-hour written exam, which assesses the doctor's basic learning and clinical knowledge.[28] The exam is held in various centers in the United Kingdom or can be taken at the British Council in such countries as Egypt, India,[29] Nigeria, Pakistan, South Africa, Sri Lanka, United Arab Emirates, and the West Indies. Overseas doctors could thus pass the first part before arriving to the United Kingdom. The second part, on the other hand, is given only at special clinical assessment centers in Britain.[30] In addition to testing clinical skills, the PLAB also measures the doctor's communication skills.[31]

In 2005, many of the doctors I spoke with had either finished the PLAB or were still stuck in one of its two stages. I listened to many stories describing the difficulties of the exam and the accompanying mandatory English language test. The preparations for the exam are laborious and time consuming. They require a full-time commitment and present a challenge for day-to-day living for an immigrant doctor. For many physicians, a source of income was crucial to survive in an expensive country like the United Kingdom. Applicants also have to pay enormous fees to take the exam—around 600 pounds, plus other hidden charges and expenses. Many doctors seeking asylum subsisted on the humble state welfare benefits offered to new arrivals. In many cases they had to use this meager sum to support their families and for everyday living expenses. Many had to find menial jobs to boost their income.

To deal with this expensive and time-consuming process, doctors strategized individually and collectively. They also mobilized personal ties in Britain and social networks from Iraq to navigate the troubles of preparing for the exam. Although some opted to stay in the capital, where most Iraqi doctors congregated, others chose a less conventional scheme. One group of twenty Iraqi doctors chose to move to Bridgend, a Welsh town of roughly 40,000 people. The Iraqi "insurgency" started after one Baghdadi doctor—an Iraqi-Briton with family connections to the town—moved in 1997.[32] His father was a renowned Iraqi physician who practiced in the United Kingdom during the 1970s, when he met and married a nurse working in the NHS. This doctor became the focal point for many of his medical colleagues from Baghdad who, upon arrival in the United Kingdom, headed to Bridgend for their asylum and career transitions. The Welsh town enjoyed a much lower cost of living. These doctors shared two large flats, living together and preparing for the exam as a group. For many it was critical to be with other colleagues for both intellectual and moral support.

Passing the PLAB test did not mean landing a position in the NHS. As one senior Iraqi consultant at the NHS explained to newly arriving compatriots, "Your CV [curriculum vitae] is your passport! It is your life and a way to impress those who would hire you here in Britain." While preparing to find a career in the NHS, then, many doctors had to apply for unpaid internships or took on locum positions at British hospitals, covering for staff shortages—the goal being to acquire "British experience" for their CVs. After 2006—with the flood of EU doctors from Greece, Poland, and Italy who, under EU labor law, required no licensing to work in Britain—these jobs also became difficult to find. More and more Iraqi doctors were struggling to even secure unpaid positions in the NHS.

One of those was Hasan, an energetic young physician who had high hopes of pursuing a career in Britain. He was the son of a well-known Iraqi doctor who had practiced in the United Kingdom during the 1960s. Hasan was married to Reem, who was also a physician. Both Hasan and Reem exemplified the complexities and sacrifices engendered in managing family life in Britain while seeking employment prospects. The two doctors lived away from their child, who was being cared for outside Britain by the wife's family. They saw each other once a week and saw their son every few months. Reem was a British citizen, born in the United Kingdom during her parents' postgraduate studies in the 1970s. After arriving in the United Kingdom, she worked in a department store for more than a year to pay government taxes and acquire a British National Insurance number—required for any paid job in the United Kingdom.

When Hasan joined his partner, she had passed the PLAB and landed an unpaid position in a hospital in Essex. After arriving in London, Hasan had had difficulty securing his licensure. He passed the English test and the two stages of the PLAB on the second try. While preparing for the exam, he worked in a private legal office translating documents from Arabic to English. It paid decently, better than the few hundred pounds he received from welfare. Recounting his predicament, he explained: "Life here is very difficult, Omar. You have rent, council tax, and various other expenses of life. I have a wife and a son, which means our expenses are huge." Hasan quit his job at the office and reverted to welfare so he could focus on his PLAB exam. After passing PLAB he tried to find a job, this time, as a medical doctor. When I met with him, he was applying for more than a hundred posts each month. It was a full-time job, he explained. Hasan was feeling drained and desperate. Our conversation then captured his general state of anger, frustration, and disappointment with the whole system. I quote at length:

> To send these applications for jobs, each week I am paying £30–40 for stamps, envelopes, and ink for the printer. The hospitals that put up these job postings are real bastards. They know most of the people who are applying are actually jobless and have no income. They require five copies

of the long application forms and five copies of your CV. They don't do the photocopying themselves because they are lazy and require from us to do all the work for them. I have to replace my inkjet after four applications, which usually costs me around £20. They also do not answer you. They write "if you don't hear from us, consider yourself not short-listed." I apply for thirty jobs each week. When I speak to the consultants in many of these hospitals they tell you that you are required to have "UK experience." I have done a one-month clinical attachment in a UK hospital, but they do not consider this "UK experience." I asked one of the consultants once if he thought that the UK experience was something "genetic" or is a form of inheritance! How can you get an experience if you cannot get a job? I told the doctor, if he thought that my father could pass this experience to me in his will, I would ask him to die soon, so I can inherit it from him! I begged him to give me a chance even for two months. He laughed. It is the chicken and the egg story. I am really waiting for a miracle to break this chain.

Beefing up one's "British experience" was one of the main paradoxes that faced Hasan and other Iraqi doctors in his situation. His sarcastic comment pointed to the British medical community's dismissal of his Iraqi training and work experience as inferior. Many other doctors internalized that feeling. One Iraqi doctor explained to his colleagues that he omitted his medical experience in Yemen because he thought that it would "look bad" on the CV that he had aimed to cultivate for a job in the United Kingdom.

For Hasan there was a self-defeating reality about the value of his training in Iraq and the reality check of trying to pursue a desirable career in Britain:

When you graduate from medical school there is usually a dream in your life that you want to pursue. But then you get shocked with the reality. Throughout medical school, I wanted to be either a vascular surgeon or urologist. But what I saw in front of me here was different. Many factors play a role, such as age, racism, and place of graduation. I started to content myself with the GP [general practitioner] line. But you know even the GP is becoming very difficult, and you have to fight for it. I had hoped that another career door would open for me. But at the end of the day if you want to live and make peace with yourself, you need to accept anything that would bring you stability. To be a consultant here is very difficult, almost impossible. I want security and safety . . . and another nationality. I want to move freely in the world. . . . I know that this will happen one day but the main question is, will you achieve that what you desired one day? We all had our ambitions; maybe if circumstances were different we would have been in another place.

The bitter disillusionment of Hasan and numerous Iraqi doctors arises from the dissonance between high expectations and daily realizations of their status as "second-class doctors" in Britain's NHS. Although this echoed with overseas doctors' historical experiences in the NHS, Iraqi doctors' lives were also shaped by their asylum predicament and their being unable to return to their home countries.

Many also considered finding alternative career paths in Britain. Sa'ad, who completed medical school in Baghdad in 1996, expressed the tensions of working as a doctor in the United Kingdom when he announced: "*El tibb ma ywakul khubuz hal ayam* [Medicine in Britain does not provide for bread these days]."

Sa'ad had worked at several jobs to support himself in the big city. "I worked in kebab places, hotels, and even as a minicab taxi driver." He was not able to land a permanent job in the NHS, which was complicated by the fact that his asylum papers were rejected. When I spoke with him, he had been appealing this ruling for the last six years. I asked Sa'ad about what he thought of the fact that it was mostly white British doctors who were to decide on the fate of overseas doctors like him. He answered: "This is their country, not mine. At this point in my life, I am just happy that I can live decently here and find a job!"

"My dream," he announced one day, "is one day to drive a Black Cab in London." "Why?" I exclaimed. "It is more fun. . . . You meet more interesting people with different stories every day. . . . You know . . . to become a Black Cab driver, you need to be a real expert in the streets of London. It takes drivers years of study to be able to pass the exam and get the license to drive a Black Cab. Can't you see that most of the drivers here are white British? Black Cab drivers are like the consultants of all the taxis in the city!"

Since the years of the mandate regime, Iraq's state medicine has been defined by its intimate relationship with the British medical enterprise. Iraqi doctors have been trained under British medical curricula and—thanks to state-building programs—have benefited over the years from specialty training in British hospitals and institutions. Despite decades of political tension between the two states, the relationship with the British enterprise was barely affected. Until the mid-1980s, successive Iraqi regimes continued to sponsor medical specialization in the United Kingdom as part of broader efforts to cultivate medical expertise and to modernize Iraqi medical science and institutions.

As asylum-seekers in the United Kingdom, Iraqi doctors confronted the limits of that historical relationship. Once agents of state modernization trained under the scientific patronage of the mandate, refugee physicians had to reconfigure their relationship with the empire, or rather its British successor regime. In Britain, these doctors struggled with asylum claims and fulfilling licensure requirements to practice and had to internalize the hierarchies and inequalities imbued in the British medical infrastructure. Iraqi doctors confronted the realities of Britain's own medical and social welfare regime—one that has been both reliant on, and partial to, its former colonies. Between asylum claims, the search for security and career entailed many compromises. Despite the reality check that many had to undergo, Iraqi doctors have come to realize that this was the state of affairs in the erstwhile imperial metropole.

British historian and diplomat Charles Webster once described the NHS as "the most civilized achievement of modern government."[33] Indeed. This achievement of civilization stands for the complex history of the empire and its various postcolonial incarnations. It is an infrastructure of state whose survival has always relied on the labor of doctors from its former colonies, which it systematically sought to disavow. Such has been the experience of many migrant doctors who have left their homes to respond to the call of the empire.

For Iraqi doctors, empire has struck once again. I saw Hasan a few times before I left London. We hung out in cafés and met often with other colleagues who updated us on their progress in the system. For our last meeting, we met in a small café in the Waterloo train station to sip coffee and eat cake. We found ourselves returning to our initial

conversation about our career dreams in the 1990s, when we were training as medical doctors in Iraq. Again he lamented his narrowing career
options, then turned his gaze on me and my decision to pursue a career
in anthropology:

> You obviously have passed through this before I did. Now you are stuck
> between two walls searching for "melon seeds in a pile of shit" [an old
> Iraqi expression]. I expected a bright future for you in medicine because
> you were one of the smarter students that I knew. I was really surprised
> when I heard that you were in a different world doing what you are doing
> now. Maybe you have discovered this fucked up situation abroad.

"Will you go back one day to Iraq?" I asked.

> Never! When we were crossing the border and my wife asked me to turn
> back for a last look, I told her, I will not. I said if we were good people
> Saddam would not have been able to rule us for more than 35 days, mind
> you 35 years. Iraq was a good medium for the growth of bacteria. I believe
> that our country will not be stable; it will always go through turmoil. This
> is final for me!

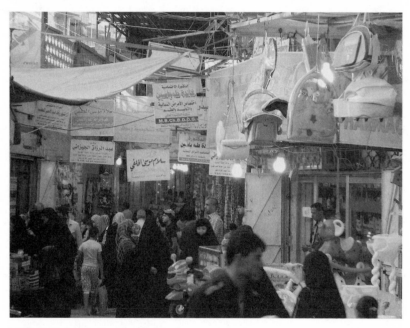

Medical clinics in a Basra market.
Photograph by Hayder Al-Mohammad

Conclusion

DURING THE SUMMER OF 2015, I received a telephone call from an old colleague from Baghdad who was planning to visit Beirut with his family for a vacation. He asked about good and decently priced hotels in the Hamra district and wanted to see me during his visit. I suggested a few places and we made plans to meet. I had not seen my friend for close to thirteen years. We lost touch after I left Iraq, but we had recently reconnected over Facebook. A month after our phone call, we met in an outdoor café. We caught up with each other's lives, spoke about the deteriorating situation in Iraq and the region, and exchanged notes about mutual friends from medical school and their whereabouts across the world. An hour later, and by sheer serendipity, three other Iraqi colleagues of ours who were coincidently in town joined us. Two were on vacation with their families. The third doctor was now himself a patient. Having been diagnosed with bone cancer, he was in Beirut for medical examinations and chemotherapy treatments.

The five of us sipped tea and smoked shisha. My colleagues exchanged notes about the best tourist sites in Beirut and good places for them and their children to spend time while in Lebanon. Soon, our conversations veered back toward work and life in Iraq.

My colleagues were all disgruntled with their jobs and the volatile security situation across the country, especially in the capital. We

exchanged stories about medical colleagues who have been killed, kidnapped for ransom, or beaten up by patients' families. We pondered
the story of one classmate who escaped his kidnappers by jumping over
rooftops in some remote neighborhood outside Baghdad. Such stories
spoke to the increasing horrors of living in Iraq as a doctor. We discussed how more and more doctors are moving out of Baghdad for work.
The irony of this situation was that doctors were now escaping to the
hinterlands, unlike earlier generations who tried to escape rural areas to
get back to Baghdad. One colleague explained that he had decided to
move to Nasiriya, the city where his wife's relatives lived. Though severely
under-resourced, the place was, he found, much safer to live and work
in than the capital. Another friend explained that he was hoping to be
transferred from Baghdad to the nearby governorate of Diyala, where
the surveillance on doctors seems less demanding. He explained that at
the capital's hospitals, the Iraqi Ministry of Health has introduced a fin-
gerprinting system to monitor doctors' movements in and out of work.
Some doctors were trying to find a way around this new restriction and
had even gone so far as paying the person in charge of the system for the
use of one of his fingers instead of their own.

My friends reported that the general public's and media's resentment against doctors seems to be on the rise. Every day there are numerous TV reports about medical errors and accusations that the country's
physicians are losing their "moral compass." Still, these problems seemed
dramatically less severed than the time of the sectarian strife in 2006 and
2007, when doctors were attacked in hospitals just because their names
betrayed their religious background. "Those were the good old days," one
of our colleagues remarked sarcastically, "when we had to carry two ID
cards, depending on the place we worked, or bought a fake ID with a
neutral name that was used by the two sides."

"I wish I had left the country a long time ago," one friend said at
some point. "I keep thinking that staying in Iraq as a doctor was the big-
gest mistake of my life."

There was a short silence. It was clear that when we all started our
medical training in the aftermath of the 1991 Gulf War, none of us had
imagined, not even in our darkest dreams, the conditions in Iraq today.
Where health care and mandatory medicine were once at the center

of governance and the state-making project, their dismemberment has characterized Iraq's ungovernability up to the present day. The breakdown of the country's medical infrastructure, the exodus of thousands of doctors, the increasing vulnerability of the figure of the physician, and the changing landscape of health-care provision inside and outside Iraq—all radically transformed the biopolitical state in Iraq.

Written against the grain of state-making accounts of Iraq, this book traces a genealogy of medicine and governance, and analyzes the historical movements and shifts that have shaped, and undermined, efforts to cultivate medicine and doctors as instruments of state making. By doing so, this book has explored how medicine and medical infrastructure have been central to the state's architecture of governance and what it has meant for this infrastructure to be targeted by decades of Western-instigated wars in the country. I have suggested that one way to understand the undermining of the state's authority in the post-1990s era, and the continual shifts and fluctuations of its governing apparatus, is to see the doctors themselves as part of a history of the making and unmaking of infrastructure. This begins to explain why the loss of so many Iraqi physicians since the 1990s has had such a huge impact not only on the material workings of the medical system itself, but also on the place medicine would come to hold in Iraq.

The current state of health and health care in Iraq needs to be situated in the aftermaths of British imperial rule and US attempts to dismantle legacies of state-making history. It reveals underlying logics of ungovernability that have persisted through these historical moments of building and destroying. Often described as the cradle of civilization, Mesopotamia, in the heart of which lies Iraq, has been central to colonial fantasies and nightmares. Since World War I, British efforts to rule Iraq have been accompanied by discourses that portrayed Iraq's territories and populations as "ungovernable"—a pathology with which imperial powers needed to reckon. From the management of the breakdown of medical infrastructure during World War I to the unintended consequences of rapid modernization under the British mandate, discourses of—and practices concerned with—Iraq's "ungovernability" often reflected the fragilities and anxieties of the colonial order. These same discourses also highlighted the importance of cultivating a medical infrastructure in response to ecological and medical uncertainties that threatened regimes of control prior to and during the British mandate. The central cog of this medical infrastructure was mandatory medicine—the platform on which the statecraft project was imagined and exercised.

The mandatory medicine experiment in Iraq emerged at a critical point in imperial history, where the British Empire was no longer able to acquire new colonies and therefore invested its efforts in state-making projects. It drew upon knowledge and expertise from both the metropole and the colonies, and improvised in the face of local and regional contingencies. The "birth" of mandatory medicine in Iraq can be traced back to the creation of Iraq's first medical school and to the country's first locally trained doctors. Mandatory medicine involved reformatting relations of science patronage that defined medical training and mobility in the region under Ottoman rule. It also defined a tradition of training Iraqi doctors that was caught up in a double movement—sending doctors to the West for training in specialized field, and deploying them to serve in the country's rural areas. This double movement caused a conundrum, as young doctors' aspirations to specialize in the British metropole was often at oddds with mandatory rural service—an obligation they frequently tried to avoid. This left large parts of the country underserved, with a concentration of doctors in major cities and provincial centers.

The mandatory medicine experiment captured the broader ethos and paradoxes of science, development, and state making during different historical moments and under different regimes of rule. In the aftermath of World War II, the fear of the spread of communist ideas and the inability to control the rising regional inequalities within the country led to the adoption of national development projects in the 1950s. These state interventions, which were meant to boost the national economy through technical fixes and to mint a new social order, were caught in the logics of urban development and rural neglect, and were instrumental in shaping the irreversible migration of rural populations to major cities. This movement conjured old and new medical discourses about unruly peasants who were redefining the urban landscape and posing a threat to its inhabitants. Ironically, it was those projects that helped trigger the 1958 revolution led by 'Abdul Karim Qasim that overthrew Iraq's British-backed monarchy.

The state's focus on medical outreach to the countryside and its impoverished population became more pronounced under succeeding governments, as medicine and housing projects became central to the state's social welfare project. The extension of state health-care was also among the central consequences of the Iran–Iraq war, with the Baʻth regime investing in primary care and mobilizing the country's female population to help improve productivity and increase reproduction. The improvement of medical and public health infrastructure during the Iran–Iraq war represented an interesting case of doing biopolitics in wartime; despite the scale of death and suffering, the state managed to expand its medical infrastructure and services. In contrast, the subsequent decades of US-led wars and Western interventions have been witness to the malicious dismemberment of Iraq's medical enterprise and the flight of the country's expert physicians.

My account of state making and unmaking in Iraq is not meant to be a comprehensive one. Instead, I have chosen the lens of a *history of the present*, piecing together the different, sometimes fragmented, evidence and sources that have allowed me to trace the complex political and social processes that shaped the country's biopolitical infrastructure since the inception of the state under the British Mandate. Furthermore, I broadened the ethnographic gaze away from Iraq by examining the experiences of Iraqi doctors in the United Kingdom, and of Iraqi patients in Lebanon, with the aim of reflecting the dynamics and reach of the dismemberment of the Iraqi state. Focusing on the institutional history of state medicine, I have suggested that the breakdown of the Iraqi state is a consequence of its entanglement in postcolonial state-making practices and the impact these practices have had on everyday social and material relations.

In light of this transnational history, my analysis of the current state of the country's health-care infrastructure allows us to go beyond simplistic and static depictions of the Iraqi state as simply a repressive entity or as a showcase of US imperial wars. Challenging historical accounts of Iraq's inherent "unruliness" under imperial forms of coercion and more recent accounts of the dismantling of the postcolonial state under the neoliberal doctrine, I have argued that the present state of governmental collapse in Iraq should be situated within alternative, yet overlapping, historical processes that transcend national borders and the periodization of colonial and postcolonial state-making.

Going beyond a contribution to Iraq's historiography, my analysis sought to situate Iraq within the history of medicine and empire. As a study in medicine and statecraft, the Iraqi case offers insights into the continuities and breaks shaping the center-periphery dynamics of science and medicine networks. I have demonstrated this by blurring the lines between Iraq's colonial and postcolonial history, and by tracing the movement of knowledge and expertise along the networks of science patronage linking Iraq and Britain. Probing the recent exodus of Iraqi doctors and their struggles to work and live in the British metropole, I have shown how the Iraqi medical establishment has been a contested domain of colonial as well as postcolonial forces. Tracing the continuities and shifts of medical training as a project of state building in Iraq, and physicians' later mass migration to the United Kingdom, I have gestured to the ways Britain's colonial legacy reverberates not only in the depletion of Iraq's medical labor force, but also in the troubled history of Britain's National Health Service.

The history of Iraq's biopolitics points to how the notion of the "ungovernable" might be a useful analytic for understanding the workings and dynamics of power. Anthropologists have often mobilized Foucault's notions of biopolitics and governmentality to rethink how state practices—such as bureaucracy and biomedical interventions—are deployed, lived, and negotiated.[1] Scholars have often looked "for signs of administrative and hierarchical rationalities that provide seemingly ordered links with the political and regulatory apparatus of a central bureaucratic state."[2] Anthropologists have furthermore focused on the state's social and territorial margins in order to discern the limits of the biopolitical state and to challenge these "parochial sightings." Building on these insights, my reading of the biopolitical state in postcolonial Iraq has found the entire state to be a margin in which the constellations of historically situated regimes of knowledge and power are continuously confronting their own limits. Central to this account is a framing of power, not as a *fait accompli*, but as a dynamic terrain of social and material life that is constantly under negotiation, forever immersed in its own contradictions and ungovernability.

My analysis of "ungovernability" in Iraq aimed to inquire into the complexities and dynamics of local and transnational regimes in shaping state authority, biopolitical practices, and citizenship. Broadly speaking, by focusing on Iraq one can begin to see how constellations of ungovernability have become amplified and instrumentalized in the ongoing US War on Terror, the breakdown of regimes across the contemporary Middle East, and the challenges the movement of refugees has posed to the European status quo. These matters speak to broader theoretical and ethnographic debates and concerns that deserve further investigation.

Wounds

The British Mandate constituted a vast historical experiment linking medicine and statecraft, resulting in a functioning biopolitical order. Political and military interventions since the 1990s have replaced that experiment with one focused on dismantling a functioning biopolitical state. The massive bombing campaigns of the Gulf War, followed by twelve years of economic sanctions, close to a decade of military occupation, and the proliferation of unruly militant groups have left hundreds of thousands of Iraqis dead and brought the country's infrastructure to ruins. Millions of Iraqis—including the country's professional classes— have been displaced both inside and outside the country. These decades of intervention have given rise to violence that continues to threaten the security of everyday life in Iraq and undermine any state-building efforts. The US occupation and its aftermath are the historical inversion of the experiment of state building that began with the British Mandate. In the dark mirror of war, American "state building" is revealed to be the dismantling of a biological and political order that was crafted in the time of the British Mandate.

Since the 1990s, this vast biological and political experiment has reflected in experiences of human suffering, the exodus of doctors, and the undermining of medical authority. But beyond this there is a more sinister story—that of the radical makeover of the nature of illness and affliction. The legacies of the biopolitical experiment initiated by sanctions and the US invasion and occupation have come to be inscribed in the traveling wounds of Iraqis seeking health care in neighboring states.[3]

The corridors of the American University of Beirut Medical Center (AUBMC) bustle with Iraqi patients and their relatives. Many have been traveling to Lebanon as frequently as once a month to receive chemotherapy, radiotherapy, or to undergo surgical procedures for war-related injuries and illnesses. All departments of this 400-bed teaching hospital have seen a rise in the numbers of Iraqis, but this is especially evident in the cancer ward. In fact, the movement of Iraqis seeking health care across regional borders has become a phenomenon shaping the trajectories of alternative modes of health-care provision. In the face of the recession and the breakdown of their state's health-care infrastructure, this mobility is what many Iraqis have come to experience as "alternative medicine."

The tens of thousands of Iraqis who travel yearly to seek care abroad are not necessarily a privileged class. Some families have sold belongings, borrowed money from friends and relatives, or mobilized other resources to deal with loved ones' life-threatening conditions. Some have visited a spate of doctors at home before coming to Beirut. Others raise concerns about being misdiagnosed before negotiating their way out of the country. Unable to restore a sense of normalcy to the country's health-care infrastructure, the Iraqi government has started to outsource treatment for its citizens to regional health-care systems. These programs, embraced after the 2003 occupation, have taken a serious hit since the Iraqi state's declaration of austerity measures in the summer of 2014 in order to shift resources to its mobilization against the so-called Islamic State. Iraqi state funds are increasingly earmarked for war injuries of military and paramilitary personnel, more and more of whom are receiving treatment in this Beirut-based hospital.

Despite budget cuts and corruption scandals, the influx of Iraqi patients to Beirut continues unabated. Beyond being a health-care infrastructure problem, Iraqi patients seem to present a clinical challenge to doctors in Lebanon. "We see many tough cases from Iraq," explained one of the AUB hospital's surgeons. "Many are suffering from very advanced and aggressive types of cancer, which we don't usually see among a younger population. We are also struggling with high rates of multidrug resistance bacteria [MDR; superbugs that defy most antibiotics] among those who are injured in suicide bombings and the ISIS war. These bugs could be transmitted to other patients. That is why we usually put Iraqis in isolation upon arrival until we confirm the microbiological status of their wounds."

This AUB surgeon's comment speaks to the complex *biosocial* ecologies of affliction in post-occupation Iraq and their regional-global reach. Since the First Gulf War, cancer deaths in Iraq have been on the rise. According to a study conducted by the University of Basra, cancer is emerging as a major cause of death in the country's southern provinces.[4] While such reports might indicate that the low survival rates of cancer patients may be due to the compromised state of oncological care,[5] it also raises many questions about the toxic legacies of war on the Iraqi population.[6] Recent scientific studies, journalistic reports, and Iraqi doctors' accounts show a substantiated association between the US military's use of pollutant munitions (e.g., depleted uranium) and the rise in congenital deformities and stillbirths in heavily bombarded areas in the southern and western parts of the country.[7] According to one of the researchers working on this phenomenon, Iraqi medical records show "the highest rate of genetic damage in any population ever studied."[8] That said, given the challenging political realities of conducting proper empirical research on the public health consequences of war in Iraq, such reports seem difficult to confirm. Previous efforts have often been hampered or muted by local and international pressure or have fallen on deaf ears around the globe.[9]

Still, this changing nature of Iraq's diseases and their ecologies seems far reaching and haunting. Beyond the reports and accounts of PTSD (post-traumatic stress disorder) among US veterans and the effects of toxic pits,[10] recent clinical studies by the US military have raised concerns about the increasing risk of US service members injured in Iraq developing MDR bacterial infections.[11] In fact, US military doctors have come to use the term *Iraqibacter* as a moniker for *Acinetobacter baumannii*—one of the superbugs that are thought to be responsible for many of the complications suffered by wounded US veterans.[12] Iraqibacter is increasingly considered a major cause of infection-related morbidity and mortality in US hospitals as well as in hospitals in conflict zones in the Middle East. Its ability to survive in hospital settings and develop rapid resistance to multiple classes of antimicrobial agents has been well documented in the literature and has received attention in recent reports.[13] Iraqibacter has been an increasing problem facing US civilian and military hospitals, due to the chain of evacuation and transport of soldiers from field hospitals back to domestic health-care facilities. Its spread from war settings in Iraq and Afghanistan has been attributed to nosocomial transmission from the increasing placement of military and civilian patients in close proximity, and to environmental contaminations at the site of injury due to skin colonization of local populations.[14] Iraqibacter seems to resist commonly used drugs, and requires the appropriation of previous generations of antibiotics that were abandoned decades ago due to their well-documented toxic side effects on the human body.[15]

The "unruly" nature of this superbug has raised many concerns among US doctors. "The bacteria pose a challenge because they have natural defenses that let them fight off many antibiotics," according to one of the US Centers for Disease Control and Prevention epidemiologists interviewed in a *New York Times* article. "And they are also good at improvising ways to outfox new drugs that are thrown at them . . . they are extremely hardy, and in one experiment proved capable of living on surfaces for up to 20 days. That makes them a menace in hospital rooms, where they can lurk on bed rails, tables and other furnishings and infect one patient after another unless every item in the room is thoroughly disinfected."[16]

While the proliferation of MDR bacteria among injured US veterans and its spread to civilian settings in the United States has been carefully documented by the US military, there is an untold story of much larger scale and magnitude. That is, the effects of such toxicity on the bodies of Iraqis exposed daily to bombing sites and on civilians across the Middle East where conflicts and injuries have become endemic. Studies are just beginning to show how widespread this pathogen is across different conflict settings in the region.[17] The high prevalence of Iraqibacter and other MDR pathogens can be attributed to the and unregulated use of broad-spectrum antibiotics in the management of battlefield patients and in local health-care facilities over decades. More specifically, in Iraq the high rates of MDR may be linked to the indirect effects of nearly a decade of international sanctions during the 1990s and the impact of this sanctions regime on antibiotic practices in the country during this period—as alluded to in the Preface to this book.

With diminishing options for effective antibiotic treatment and the persistence of regional conflicts, the proliferation of MDR represents a global health problem with serious repercussions. Given the protracted nature of conflicts in this region, the fragmentation of health-care systems, and the dire prospects of injured patients and refugees, MDR contributes to the present and future burdens of war injuries. Furthermore, as MDR becomes an endemic phenomenon, hospital settings are increasingly becoming dangerous and toxic places for care. Clinical and social science research will need to better understand such long-term consequences of war, consequences Iraqis will have to face and negotiate in the face of the changing biosocial realities of everyday life.

The Iraq experiment seems to have conditioned an ecology of state collapse that has spread, like a pathogen, to states elsewhere in the region, and has the potential of spreading even farther under the guise of the global War on Terror. Symptomatic of this ecology is the breakdown of once robust health-care systems, like the one in Iraq. Whether this collapse has been part of systematic efforts to dismantle the state and render life ungovernable, or merely a by-product of contingencies such as Western powers' ignorance, disorganization, and bad faith, is not a question that can be answered here. It is ironic, however, how—after Iraq's decades-long struggle to establish and improve a national health-care infrastructure—the unusually muscular afflictions suffered by Iraqis today echo the orientalizing pathologies that the first generation of British Indian army officers ascribed to the land they would occupy. Depictions of a toxic environment riddled with tropical maladies have been superseded by clinical reports of a spike in cancer rates and the spread of Iraqibacter, both formed in the crucible of international sanctions, conquest, and occupation.

There is a cruel symmetry in this imperial legacy.

Reference Matter

Notes

Introduction

1. Dewachi et. al., "Changing Therapeutic Geographies of the Iraq and Syria Wars."

2. See Paley, "Iraqi Hospitals Are War's New 'Killing Fields'," on the spiraling sectarian violence in Baghdad between 2006 and 2007, and its implications for the country's health-care system. During these turbulent years, militias affiliated with the Ministry of Health kidnapped, imprisoned, and executed doctors and patients inside hospitals and government buildings. Militia members used ambulances to abduct citizens and converted the basement of the Ministry of Health into a torture chamber.

3. Al-Auwsi, "Iraq's Doctors Are Subject to Humiliation and Murder."

4. Al-Kindi, "Violence against Doctors in Iraq."

5. Al-Auwsi, "Iraq's Doctors Are Subject to Humiliation and Murder."

6. BBC, "Iraqi Doctors to Be Allowed Guns."

7. Burnham, Lafta, and Doocy, "Doctors Leaving 12 Tertiary Hospitals in Iraq, 2004–2007."

8. My understanding of the connections among medicine, power, and state making draws on the insights and analysis of biopolitics and governmentality by Michel Foucault, see Foucault, "The Politics of Health in the Eighteenth Century"; Foucault, *Security, Territory, Population*; Foucault, *Society Must Be Defended*. Anthropologists and historians of medicine have used Foucault's analysis to understand how science, medicine, and bureaucracy have been instrumentalized as regimes of government in colonial and postcolonial contexts, as well as in Western and non-Western settings. See Anderson, *Colonial Pathologies*; Arnold, *Warm Climates and Western Medicine*; Comaroff, "The Diseased Heart of Africa"; Stoler, *Race and the Education of Desire*; Brotherton, *Revolutionary Medicine*; Nguyen, *The Republic of Therapy*. Foucault proposed that one of the main mutations that shaped Western political organization during the eighteenth and nineteenth centuries was the increasing incorporation of life processes in the strategization and operation of state apparatus and institutions—what he called biopolitics or biopower. For Foucault, biopolitics is simply population politics (Fassin, "Another Politics of Life Is Possible"), seen, for example, in the rise of public health sciences, the management of epidemics and

endemics, and urban planning and policing. Governmentality—defined as the conduct of conduct and associated with the rise of such biopolitics—denotes specific relations and technologies of power "linked to the emergence of the modern state, the political figure of the 'population', and the constitution of the economy as a specific domain of reality" (Lemke, *Foucault, Governmentality, and Critique*, 88). For Foucault, the effects of these technologies and techniques of governance fundamentally act on the body and its environment through discipline and control of the biological and social processes and relations of individuals and collectives—both within confined spaces and out in open territories. These are not necessarily repressive forms of power that govern through "domination," rather productive ones "dispersed through society, inherent in social relationships, embedded in a network of practices, institutions, and technologies—operating on all of the 'micro-levels' of everyday life" (Pylypa, "Power and Bodily Practice"). Within such a conception, power's main rationale and effect are the governing of "life itself" (Rabinow and Rose, "Biopower Today"; Rose, *The Politics of Life Itself*). In exploring the relationship between governance and life, I take the interpretation of Thomas Lemke regarding Foucault's conceptualization of biopolitics, where "life denotes neither the basis nor the object of politics. Instead, it presents a border to politics—a border that should be simultaneously respected and overcome, one that seems to be both natural and given but also artificial and transformable" (Lemke, *Biopolitics*, 4–5).

9. I take my cue from anthropological work that has examined the critical role of medical doctors in the broader politics of state making and transformations. See Adams, *Doctors for Democracy*; Iliffe, *East African Doctors*; Wendland, *A Heart for the Work*; Good, *American Medicine*.

10. For examples of the consequences of neoliberalization on health care, see Kim et al., *Dying for Growth*; Han, *Life in Debt*; Keshavjee, *Blind Spot*; Farmer et al., *Reimagining Global Health*; Biehl and Petryna, *When People Come First*; Prince and Marsland, *Making and Unmaking Public Health in Africa*.

11. Many scholars have problematized positioning neoliberal logic as a universalizing force and have shown instead the intricate complexities and role of historical and local forces in shaping state practices across the globe. See Amar, *The Security Archipelago*; Collier, *Post-Soviet Social*; Ong and Collier, *Global Assemblages* for examples.

12. Collier, *Post-Soviet Social*.

13. Petryna, *When Experiments Travel*.

14. Nguyen, *The Republic of Therapy*.

15. Redfield, *Life in Crisis*.

16. Biehl, *Vita*.

17. Povinelli, *Economies of Abandonment*.

18. Recent accounts about war and violence in the Middle East have suggested that we have entered into a new era of contemporary warfare where military and humanitarian interventions are becoming increasingly intertwined. The efforts to rule through the media-

tion of military and humanitarian interventions are contained within technologies and techniques of governance that aims to "calculate the effects of violence and . . . harness its consequences." As Eyal Weizman has poignantly argued, the will to govern under such logics is "grounded in the very ability to count, measure, balance and act on these calculations" (Weizman, *The Least of All Possible Evils,* 17). He further argues, "Inversely to make oneself ungovernable, one must make oneself incalculable, immeasurable, uncountable" (Ibid.) As I will show later, I present a different framework and genealogy of ungovernability, one that is tied to colonial history and framed as internal to the workings of regimes of power rather than being constituted in opposition to it.

19. In his famous piece on necropolitics, Achille Mbembe uses the First Gulf War as an example of infrastructural warfare where high-tech weaponry is employed in the interest of "shutting down the enemy's life support" and doing "enduring damage of civilian life." He argues that under such conditions of warfare, "Weapons are deployed in the interest of maximum destruction of persons and the creation of *death-worlds*" as "vast populations are subjected to conditions of life conferring upon them the status of *living dead"* (Mbembé, "Necropolitics," 40).

20. The impact of the war and sanctions on Iraq's public health and medical infrastructure was much greater than that of other states under economic embargo in the 1990s, such as Cuba. In stark contrast to Cuba's ability to maintain the integrity of its health-care infrastructure under sanctions, the First Gulf War and the consequences of sanctions on state medicine fomented infrastructure breakdown in Iraq. For the consequences of the economic sanctions and the collapse of the Soviet Union during the 1990s, see Brotherton, *Revolutionary Medicine.*

21. Gordon, "Economic Sanctions and Global Governance: The Case of Iraq."

22. For the most comprehensive study of the UN Security Council sanctions in Iraq, see Gordon, *Invisible War.*

23. Gordon, *Invisible War.*

24. On the direct effects of sanctions on Iraqi society see Hall and Olafimihan, "A Dose of the UN's Medicine"; Ascherio et al., "Effect of the Gulf War on Infant and Child Mortality in Iraq"; Gordon, *Invisible War*; Court, "Iraq Sanctions Lead to Half a Million Child Deaths"; Garfield, "Morbidity and Mortality among Iraqi Children from 1990 through 1998."

25. There has been a wide range of Western media articles that have used the term *ungovernable* to describe the condition of violence and the failure to establish order in Iraq. See Reynolds, "Iraq the Ungovernable"; Ulhmann, "Iraq Close to Ungovernable"; Leader, "Ungoverned and Ungovernable."

26. Bouillon, "Iraq's State-Building Enterprise"; Dodge, *Inventing Iraq*; Fromkin, *A Peace to End All Peace.*

27. Dodge, *Inventing Iraq.*

28. Davis, *Memories of State*. According to Davis, Iraq has been torn between two models of nationalism—pan-Arab and Iraqi. The absence of an acceptable model of political community has led to the failure to establish a collective identity.

29. Khoury, *Iraq in Wartime*.

30. Makiya, *Republic of Fear*; Sassoon, *Saddam Hussein's Ba'th Party*.

31. Farouk-Sluglett and Sluglett, "The Historiography of Modern Iraq."

32. Ahram, "Iraq in the Social Sciences," 251.

33. Ibid., 251.

34. Ibid., 253.

35. An exception to this dearth of critical work on Iraq has been the writings of anthropologist Hayder al-Mohammed, whose analysis of everyday life in post-occupation Basra has opened new avenues for theoretical and empirical research on the country. Based on prolonged ethnographic fieldwork, al-Mohammed has efficiently shown how—in the context of deterioration of security, militia kidnappings, and breakdown of the country's infrastructures—everyday life in Iraq is predicated on ethical modes of sociality and dwelling that contrast with the somewhat flat representations in media and academia of social life in the country. See al-Mohammad, "A Kidnapping in Basra"; al-Mohammad and Peluso, "Ethics and the 'Rough Ground' of the Everyday"; al-Mohammad, "Ordure and Disorder"; al-Mohammad, "Towards an Ethics of Being-With"; al-Mohammad, "'You Have Car Insurance, We Have Tribes.'"

36. The impact of the 2003 invasion on the destruction of the country's archive has been well documented (see Khoury, "Iraq's Lost Cultural Heritage"). Since 2003, however, there have been two main archival collections that have become available to researchers in the West. The first is the Saddam Hussein Regime Collection, housed at the National Defense University's Conflict Record Research Center (CRRC) in Washington, DC. The second is the Ba'th Party Records collection, housed at the Hoover Institution archive at Stanford University. These two collections have been highly politicized, as they were seized and confiscated by the US military and transported to the United States. See Montgomery's description in "Immortality in the Secret Police Files."

37. In lieu of the methodological challenges of such an undertaking, I have used myriad primary and secondary sources in English and Arabic to trace this history. I examined historical documents and collections at international universities and Iraqi research centers, and I conducted scores of interviews with different generations of Iraqi doctors and government employees both in Iraq and in exile. I read numerous autobiographical accounts of Iraqi doctors and other civil servants, as well as local historiographies of its health-care system. I have used accounts from different technical reports and academic articles from the periods I covered that pertained to the subject of my analysis. During my residence in the United Kingdom (2005–2006), I spent most of my time in London living with and interacting with different generations of Iraqi doctors and expats. The state of the country's archive necessitated that I triangulate any available material to make better

sense of the history, and I anchored my interpretation of the data in my own personal experience of growing up and living in Iraq for twenty-five years.

38. Taussig, *Shamanism, Colonialism, and the Wild Man*, xiii.

39. There is a long history of philosophical thought that draws from Kant, Nietzsche, Weber, Marx, and the Frankfurt school that has addressed internal dialectics of power. See for example Adorno and Horkheimer, *Dialectic of Enlightenment*.

40. Scott, *Weapons of the Weak*; Scott, *The Art of Not Being Governed*.

41. Here I take my cue from recent critical work in the anthropology of medicine that has problematized the notion of culture and suggested alternate frameworks that pay more attention to the materiality of the body proper and the way "culture, history, politics, and biology (environmental and individual) are inextricably entangled and subject to never-ending transformations" (Lock and Nguyen, *An Anthropology of Biomedicine*, 1).

42. Arnold, "'Illusory Riches'"; Anderson, *The Cultivation of Whiteness*; Anderson, *Colonial Pathologies*; Mbembe, *On the Postcolony*; Moulin, "Tropical without the Tropics"; Said, *Orientalism*. Regarding nineteenth-century Europe, see Pick, *Faces of Degeneration*.

43. Arnold, *Colonizing the Body*.

44. Anderson, *The Cultivation of Whiteness*; Vaughan, "Health and Hegemony."

45. Anderson, *Colonial Pathologies*.

46. Harrison, "Chapter 5, Wonder and Pain, Mesopotamia November 1914–May 1916."

47. Great Britain. Colonial Office, "Mesopotamia: Handbook Prepared under the Direction of the Historical Section of the Foreign Office–No. 63," 7.

48. The development of the field of tropical medicine in the West is one example of the history of colonial medicine. Tropical medicine has been linked to a 400-year-old history of European colonial encounters. It emerged as a set of knowledge and practices in the colony that were concerned with ailments and therapies specific to the "tropics" and other hot climates in Asia, America, and Africa. As others have argued, tropical medicine played an important role in shaping Western perceptions of distant lands and populations. It has also been instrumentalized in the control of local populations and in ensuring the survival of Europeans in alien environments. Moulin, "Tropical without the Tropics."

49. In other settings, tropical conditions challenged the integrity of the "white" colonial body, and discourses about its imminent physical breakdown pointed to the limits of regimes of control. See Anderson, *Colonial Pathologies*; Anderson, *The Cultivation of Whiteness*; Rogaski, *Hygienic Modernity*.

50. See Anderson, *Colonial Pathologies*; Anderson, "Making Global Health History"; Arnold, *Colonizing the Body*; Stoler, *Race and the Education of Desire*; Rabinow, *French Modern*.

51. Anderson, "Making Global Health History," 381.

52. Mitchell, *Rule of Experts*.

53. It was not until decades after the inauguration of the first medical school that the Iraqi state invested in the creation of local schools to train other professions in the sciences of engineering.

54. Das, *Critical Events*.

55. During the 1950s, the writings of Iraqi sociologist Ali al-Wardi captured the tensions of statecraft and development imperatives. This will be covered in more detail in Chapter Five of this book.

56. Sayegh, *Child Survival in Wartime*.

57. In thinking of "doctors as infrastructure," I here draw insights from the work of AbdouMaliq Simone and his analysis of marginal populations in South Africa. See Simone, "People as Infrastructure: Intersecting Fragments in Johannesburg." I further draw on anthropological insights about the workings of infrastructure as structures, networks, and affects embedded in human and material relations of power and circulation. See Larkin, "The Politics and Poetics of Infrastructure" and the curated collection on "Infrastructure" in *Cultural Anthropology*, edited by Jessica Lockrem and Adonia Lugo.

Chapter 1

1. Great Britain. Foreign Office. Historical Section. "Mesopotamia: Handbook Prepared under the Direction of the Historical Section of the Foreign Office–No. 63," 1.

2. Also called the Indian Expeditionary Force D (IEF D).

3. See Sluglett, *Britain in Iraq*.

4. For a discussion on tensions between Britain's Cairo Bureau and Indian government and the change in policy regarding its plans in Mesopotamia, see Sluglett, *Britain in Iraq, 1914–1932*; Wilson, *Loyalties Mesopotamia 1914–1917*.

5. Linebagh, "May Day at Kut and Kenthal."

6. "The Campaign in Iraq: A paper read before the Hunterian Society St George's Hospital on Feb 26th 1920," 2–3.

7. Morris, *Farewell the Trumpets*, 171.

8. See the discussion on the breakdown of the medical provisions during the Mesopotamian campaign in Harrison, "Chapter 5, Wonder and Pain, Mesopotamia November 1914–May 1916."

9. As medical historian Mark Harrison has shown, the medical services and hygiene regulations of the British military were boosted across both the Western and non-Western fronts as medical organization was becoming integral to the management of the troops' health and morale. Harrison, *The Medical War*.

10. "The Campaign in Iraq," 3.

11. Headrick, *The Tools of Empire*.

12. For more on the expedition, see Chesney, *The Expedition for the Survey of the Rivers Euphrates and Tigris*; Chesney, *Narrative of the Euphrates Expedition Carried on by Order*

of the British Government during the Years 1835, 1836 and 1837; Chesney, "Reports on the Navigation of the Euphrates."

13. Great Britain. Foreign Office. Historical Section, "Mesopotamia: Handbook Prepared under the Direction of the Historical Section of the Foreign Office–No. 63."

14. Saleh, *Britain and Mesopotamia (Iraq to 1914)*, 179.

15. Lynch, "Note Accompanying a Survey of the Tigris between Ctesiphone and Mosul"; Jones, "Journal of a Steam Voyage to the North of Baghdad, in April, 1846"; Loftus, "Notes of a Journey from Baghdad to Busrah, with Descriptions of Several Chaldaean Remains."

16. Heffernan, "Geography, Cartography and Military Intelligence."

17. Lynch, "Note Accompanying a Survey of the Tigris between Ctesiphone and Mosul," 442.

18. Harrison, *The Medical War*, 223.

19. "The Campaign in Iraq," 6.

20. Harrison, "Chapter 5, Wonder and Pain, Mesopotamia November 1914–May 1916."

21. Sinderson, *Ten Thousand and One Nights; Memories of Iraq's Sherifian Dynasty*, 25.

22. Moulin, "Tropical without the Tropics," 161.

23. "The Campaign in Iraq," 7.

24. Sinderson, *Ten Thousand and One Nights*, 32.

25. The British army also tried to regulate the entry and exit to the *Kalachiyyeh*, the local brothels, on the main street to minimize the risks of syphilis among the troops. They used signs written in English, Arabic, and Urdu to block one of the two existing exits. See Baghdadi, *Baghdad Fi al'Ishrinat* [Baghdad in the Twenties].

26. Baghdad boil, or leishmaniasis, is a parasitic disease caused by a bite of the female sand fly, which is tiny enough to pass through a mosquito net. It starts as a slow-growing wart, usually on exposed parts of the body, such as the face or the forearms. It has a tendency to break and suppurate, and if left alone, the condition subsides gradually in about seven months, leaving a very evident scar on its victim. In cities like Baghdad at the time, many local inhabitants were actually identified through their scar, which they most usually acquired when they were young. Still today, it is commonly referred to in Iraq as *Habat Baghdad*, or Baghdad boil, indicating its endemic nature in that city.

27. Arnold, *Warm Climates and Western Medicine*, 10.

28. As David Arnold has shown, concerns of the role of climate in the etiology of diseases continued to shape the discourses of tropical medicine in many colonial settings during and after the proliferation of the germ theory.

29. Sinderson, *Ten Thousand and One Nights*, 31.

30. Ibid.

31. "The Campaign in Iraq," 12–13.

32. Ibid., 12.

33. Ibid.13.

34. Ibid., 11.

35. Ibid., 14.

36. Sinderson, *Ten Thousand and One Nights*, 28.

37. In his work on early colonial narratives about Australia, Warwick Anderson shows the role of medicine in the production of a notion of whiteness through acclimatization narratives of British bodies to their new harsh environment. Anderson explains that discourses about acclimatization revealed the way white colonial settlers attempted "to match their personal sense of bodily terrain with their novel environment, adjusting their diet, clothing, housing, and physical activity in order to establish a harmony of individuality and circumstances." Anderson, *The Cultivation of Whiteness*, 11.

38. Sinderson, "Some Recollections of Iraq, 1918–1946," 221.

Chapter 2

1. Quoted in Abélès, *The Politics of Survival*, 33.

2. Westrate, *The Arab Bureau*.

3. Great Britain. "Special Report by His Majesty's Government in the United Kingdom of Great Britain and Northern Ireland to the Council of the League of Nations on the Progress of Iraq during the Period 1920–1931," no. 58, 64.

4. From the Proclamation of Baghdad, issued to the inhabitants of Baghdad on March 19, 1917, by Lieutenant General Sir Stanley Maude.

5. On the historical significance of the Financial Crisis of the British Empire, see Arrighi, "Hegemony Unravelling-1."

6. Higgins, "World War I and Its Effects on British Financial Institutions."

7. Sluglett, *Britain in Iraq*.

8. The Arab Bureau was a section of Britain's Cairo Intelligence Department during World War I and was very influential in shaping its policies in the post-Ottoman provinces during the pre-Mandate years. See Westrate, *The Arab Bureau*.

9. Lawrence, "T. E. Lawrence to Lord Curzon." In this letter on September 27, 1919, to Lord Curzon, British Foreign Secretary and former Viceroy of India, T. E. Lawrence explained: "My own ambition is that the Arabs should be our first brown dominion, and not our last brown colony."

10. Class A included Iraq, Palestine, Transjordan Emirate, and Syria (including Lebanon); Class B included Ruanda-Urundi, Tanganyika, Cameroon, and Togoland; Class C included New Guinea, Nauru, Samoa, South Pacific Mandate, and South West Africa. Consequently, indirect rule varied according to the level of control held by the mandatory power over a territory.

11. Article 22, *The League of Nations in Retrospect*.

12. Sluglett, *Britain in Iraq*, 5–6.

13. Mesopotamian Expeditionary Force, "Preliminary Scheme of Civil Medical Provision for Mesopotamia."

14. Ibid., 2.

15. Ibid., 2–3.

16. Ibid., 2.

17. Sinderson, *Ten Thousand and One Nights*, 33.

18. The argument of the two doctors resonated with postwar calls in Britain to reform the country's fragmented health services. Such debates, which later contributed to the formation of Britain's National Health Service (NHS) in 1948, were being resisted by the country's affluent medical doctors. See Porter, *Health, Civilization, and the State*.

19. Sinderson, *Ten Thousand and One Nights*, 34.

20. Both Arabic words come from the same root, h.k.m.

21. It has been suggested that Iraq was central to the development of Britain's strategies of air policing after World War I. Although the bombing of tribes has been a common practice, it has been suggested that this was the first time in history that aerial photography was used to awe the locals into submission. On air policing see Omissi, *Air Power and Colonial Control*. On the centrality of air policing in Iraq, see Dodge, *Inventing Iraq*.

22. The conception of the NHS as a model of state medicine faced strong resistance from many medical professionals and politicians from the Conservative Party. Medical professionals in particular saw these policies as a government infringement upon the autonomy and the authority of local decentralized structures of philanthropy and medical aid. In Britain, this tension between the reach of central government and the autonomy of local governments continued to shape political debates throughout the first half of the twentieth century, hindering the complete realization of state medicine. See Porter, *Health, Civilization, and the State*.

23. Porter, "How Did Social Medicine Evolve, and Where Is It Heading?"; Porter, *Health, Civilization, and the State*; Porter, *The History of Public Health and the Modern State*.

24. In Britain, politicians such as Edwin Chadwick and medical doctors such as John Simon were instrumental in centralizing the role of medicine as an administrative instrument of the state in the regulations of populations' health. See Porter, *Health, Civilization, and the State*.

25. This urban squalor was a product of the rapid industrialization of British society during the eighteenth and nineteenth centuries. See Porter, *Health, Civilization, and the State*.

26. Stedman Jones, *Outcast London*.

27. Porter, *Health, Civilization, and the State*.

28. Mesopotamian Expeditionary Force, "Mesopotamia Civil Medical Service."

29. Ibid.

30. On the social and medical history of the Anglo-Boer wars, see van Heyningen, *The Concentration Camps of the Anglo-Boer War*.

31. Tripp, *A History of Iraq*.

32. Sluglett, *Britain in Iraq, 1914–1932*; Wilson, *Loyalties Mesopotamia 1914–1917*; Dodge, *Inventing Iraq*; Main, *Iraq from Mandate to Independence*.

33. Lane, "Administration Report of the Health Department 1919–1920."

34. These included one chemist, seventeen civil surgeons, one dental surgeon, one medical officer of health, one ophthalmic surgeon, one pathologist, one lady doctor, twelve nursing sisters, four sanitary inspectors, and two other non-Gazetted staff. Ibid.

35. Identifying medical administration with security underscored that intimate connection between health care and policing. See Foucault, *Security, Territory, Population*.

36. As a Christian from Mosul, he was seen as someone bringing more diversity to the newly elected cabinet. The first cabinet included a number of minorities representing the diverse constituency of the imagined Iraqi cultural landscape.

37. The publication of these reports ranged from 1918–1927.

38. Heggs, "Annual Report of the Health Department for the Year 1921," 1.

39. Ibid., 2.

40. Ibid., 1.

41. Ibid., 2.

42. Ibid., 2.

43. Ibid., 2.

44. The word *moral* here represents a normative sense of good or bad morals. It refers to individuals' manners and general behavior within society. The use of this term here spells out the obvious regulatory-political dimension of public health, which is not merely concerned with prevention and treatment of physical ailments, but also with the regulation, management, and attainment of good moral conduct. The formulation of moral well-being as part of public health is reminiscent of Foucault's notion of governmentality as the conduct of conduct. See Inda, *Anthropologies of Modernity*.

45. Heggs, "Annual Report of the Health Department for the Year 1921."

46. Porter, *Health, Civilization, and the State*; Porter, *The History of Public Health and the Modern State*.

47. I am here referring to the sociological concept developed by Robert Merton. See Merton, "The Unanticipated Consequences of Purposive Social Action." See also other elaborations on the notion in Farmer et al., *Reimagining Global Health*.

48. The city is also known in Persian as Khorramshahr. The city was central to the start of the Iraq–Iran war in the 1980s, as will be discussed in Chapter Six.

49. Government of 'Iraq, "Annual Report of the Health Department for the Years 1923–1924," 10.

50. Al-Witri, *Health Services in Iraq*.

51. Great Britain. Colonial Office, "Report by His Majesty's Government on the Administration of 'Iraq for the Period April, 1923–December, 1924," 84–85.

52. Government of 'Iraq, "Annual Report of the Health Department for the Years 1923–1924," 10.

53. The cholera vaccine was pioneered by W. M. Haffkine during the 1890s in India, and had been controversial in scientific and political debates during colonial rule. See the debate on the vaccine in British medical journals: "Inoculations Against Cholera in India," *The British Medical Journal* (1895) 735–739; Haffkine, "A Lecture: Preventive Inoculation Against Cholera in India," *The Lancet* (1895) 1555–1556. See also Arnold, "Cholera and Colonialism in British India."

54. Arnold, "Cholera and Colonialism in British India."

55. Great Britain. Colonial Office, "The Administration of 'Iraq" 1923–1924, 79.

56. Ibid, 88.

57. As late as the 1930s, the Indian government categorically rejected the use of the vaccine on Hindu pilgrims who annually descended on the Ganges in Allahabad, as the political atmosphere of civil disobedience and tensions between the British and the Congress Party were rising. See Arnold, *Colonizing the Body*.

Chapter 3

1. Lane, "Administration Report of the Health Department 1919–1920," 2.

2. Rogan, *The Fall of the Ottomans.*

3. On the administration of Tanzimat in Iraq, see Cetinsaya, *The Ottoman Administration of Iraq, 1890–1908.* For a general history of Tanzimat under the Ottoman state, see Quataert, *The Ottoman Empire, 1700–1922*; Hanioğlu, *A Brief History of the Late Ottoman Empire*; Engelhardt et al., *La Turquie et le Tanzimât*; Ma'oz, *Ottoman Reform in Syria and Palestine, 1840–1861*; Fortna, *Imperial Classroom.*

4. Fahmy, *All the Pasha's Men.*

5. Ibid.

6. The Ottomans eventually established another medical school, which taught medicine in Turkish. These two schools were united and the language of instruction became Turkish.

7. Fahmy, *All the Pasha's Men.*

8. Kâhya and Erdemir, *Medicine in the Ottoman Empire.*

9. One of the main consequences of modernizing professional education was the rise of nationalist sentiment and movements persuaded by the history of social, political, and cultural transformations in Europe during the nineteenth century. Influenced by the ideas and models of secular nation-states in Europe, doctors became critical of the political and cultural organization of the Ottoman state and demanded further political and cultural reform. As a result, Ottoman medical associations became beacons for the Turkish nationalist movement. These movements would be instrumental in catalyzing the later fall of the empire after the end of World War I. On Turkish nationalism and the

fall of the Ottoman Empire, see Arai, *Turkish Nationalism in the Young Turk Era*; Haddad and Ochsenwald, *Nationalism in a Non-National State*; Kayali, *Arabs and Young Turks*.

10. Missionary activities in Mesopotamia were limited to French, German, and British groups that established a number of schools in the three cities of Mosul, Baghdad, and Basra. Few medical missionary doctors established clinics with the aim of reaching out to the local population. Many of these activities were put on hold immediately after the start of World War I in 1914.

11. Tibawi, *American Interests in Syria 1800–1901*, 203.

12. The exam was offered exclusively in Turkish at the Imperial School of Medicine in Constantinople. Daniel Bliss, then the president of the Protestant College in Beirut, made a trip to Constantinople to negotiate a form of accreditation and logistics for the licensure process. His trip failed to produce anything beyond coverage of travel expenses for doctors to the metropole. In later years, he managed to convince the education board in Constantinople to send examiners from the Imperial School to hold these exams annually in Beirut. See Tibawi, *American Interests in Syria 1800–1901*.

13. In her work on colonial medicine in Sudan, historian Heather Bell demonstrates how a good number of these graduates from Syria's two missionary universities, which included Lebanon, filled the junior ranks of the Egyptian army's medical corps and the British-controlled Sudan Defense Force, created during Anglo-Egyptian rule in Sudan (1899–1956). British officials and local Sudanese used the term *Syrian doctors* to refer to physicians trained in Beirut (then part of the Ottoman Syria province). As Bell shows, this relationship with the Syrian doctors was "structured by practical, economic and political consideration, and was always informed by racial perceptions." See Bell, "Frontiers of Medicine in the Anglo-Egyptian Sudan, 1899–1940."

14. Heggs, "Annual Report of the Health Department for the Year 1921," Appendix C.

15. Al-Samara'i, *Hadeeth Al-Thamaneen* [A Conversation at Eighty], Volume 4, 273.

16. Ibid.

17. Isaacs, "Britain's Contribution to Medicine and the Teaching of Medicine in Iraq," 24.

18. Al-Damalouji, *al-Kuliyyah al-Tibyyah al-Malakiyyah al-'Iraqiyah* [The Iraqi Royal College of Medicine], *193*.

19. Ibid.

20. Sluglett, *Britain in Iraq, 1914–1932*.

21. This was a more general imperial British educational policy in India and other colonies, which seemed to have shaped British education policy in Iraq under the mandate; see Sluglett, *Britain in Iraq, 1914–1932*, Chapter 8; Whitehead, *Colonial Educators*. Similar anxieties were also recorded in British India in the early nineteenth century. In his seminal work on the state of medicine in India, Arnold, *Colonizing the Body*, pages 54–55, shows how prior to 1835 there was an active project of training local Indian doctors in Western medical texts translated to vernacular languages. This project also

entailed the use of elements of Indian medicine incorporated into the teaching of local doctors. The project was later abandoned and was replaced by Western medicine taught in English. Another comparative perspective is that of the training of nurses in the Philippines under American colonialism. Choy, *Empire of Care*, shows how American training of local nurses was an "integral part of nursing students' curriculum, one which represented one of the unique aspects of American colonial education in general and medical education in particular," 43–44.

22. See Sluglett, *Britain in Iraq*, 194. One of the main fears of the British was the rising Bolshevik influence that was gaining ground among many young, educated, middle-class citizens.

23. It is important here to note that Iraqi elites at the time did not subscribe to one strand of Arab nationalism. These terms were very much in flux and were continuously shaped by different political, ideological, social, and personal interests.

24. See Sluglett, *Britain in Iraq*, Chapter 2, on the negotiation and correspondence between Faisal and the British government regarding the Anglo-Iraqi treaty.

25. Sluglett, *Britain in Iraq, 1914–1932*, 43.

26. For a comprehensive biography of Faisal, see Allawi, *Faisal I of Iraq*.

27. Many of these educators were part of decades of Arab intellectual revival during the late nineteenth and early twentieth century. For a history and discussion on the Arab revival or *al-Nahda*, see Elshakry, *Reading Darwin in Arabic, 1860–1950*; Patel, *The Arab Nahdah*; Pormann, "The Arab 'Cultural Awakening (Nahda),' 1870–1950, and the Classical Tradition."

28. Al-Husri, *Muthakarati Fi Al-'Iraq* [My Memoirs in Iraq], 73–74.

29. According to al-Husri, the three main state high schools in Iraq offered only four years of non-differentiated science and literature paths. He believed that the teaching of the natural sciences was still very weak and required further development.

30. Simon, *Iraq between the Two World Wars*, 76.

31. Sluglett, *Britain in Iraq, 1914–1932*, 201.

32. Al-Husri, *Muthakarati Fi al-'Iraq* [My Memoirs in Iraq], 66–68.

33. Ibid., 76–77.

34. Al-Samara'i, *Hadeeth al-Thamaneen*, Volume 4, 274–275.

35. According to the British version of the story, Farrell seemed to have resigned after the appointment of al-Husri as the director-general of education. According to the al-Husri account, he managed to convince Faisal to persuade the civil commissioner, Percy Cox, to transfer Farrell back to India. Subsequently, Farrell served under the director-general of education in Palestine. See Sluglett, *Britain in Iraq, 1914–1932*, 200–201.

36. Government of 'Iraq, "Annual Report of the Health Department for the Years 1923–1924," 4.

37. Sinderson, *Ten Thousand and One Nights*, 109.

38. Law of Medical Practice in Iraq. See Hallinan, "Report of Inspector-General, The Iraqi Health Services for the Years 1925 & 1926," 101.

39. Ibid.

40. Ibid., 102.

41. The constitution called for a bicameral parliament whose lower house, *Majlis al-Nuwwab* or Chamber of Deputies, would be "elected," based on Sluglett, *Britain in Iraq, 1914–1932*, 201. Supported by British policy of the mandate, however, the "elected" members of the parliament were chosen through indirect ballots rather than direct suffrage. As a result, the British were able to pack the parliament with tribal sheikhs and town politicians who were sympathetic to them during the 1920 revolt; see Haj, *The Making of Iraq, 1900–1963*. The upper house, *Majlis al-'A'yan* or the Council of Senates, was appointed directly by the king. In effect, members of both houses were more or less selected rather than elected. This continued until 1952 when indirect elections ended formally.

42. These doctors were Sa'ib Shawkat, Tawfeeq Rushdi, and Hashim al-Witri, all of whom had trained in Istanbul and returned to Iraq after the war.

Chapter 4

1. Al-Samara'i, *Hadeeth al-Thamaneen* [A Conversation at Eighty] Volume 1, 120–121.

2. Ibid., 132.

3. More autobiographies have been published over the past few decades than in the decades after its inauguration. These accounts have been written with an air of nostalgia to a "better" past, celebrating the rigor and quality of education at the school during these years. For many of these doctors, these were the days of the *ingleez*, the English, who dominated the teaching faculty and presented a more serious and prestigious training.

4. Anthropologist Michael Fischer argues for the use of autobiography as a "vehicle for access for anthropological investigation;" Fischer, *Emergent Forms of Life and the Anthropological Voice*, 183. For Fischer, the autobiography is a methodological tool layered with the possibility and multiplicity of voices. It is a window into various cultural processes, such as compositions of identities and dialogic relations of difference, providing a comparison and a cross-cultural critique for articulation of emotions, self, and agency. For Fischer this allows an insight into not only how these articulations work in "alternative moral traditions" but also how these moral traditions themselves emerge through these same articulations.

5. Despite the expansion of Iraq's unified education curricula over the 1920s, there were, still, only a few students who had graduated with a national baccalaureate.

6. Interview with Sa'ib Shawkat, one of the first teachers of the school and a member of the College Selection Committee. See Fkaiki, *Tareekh A'lam al-Tibb al-'Iraqi al-Hadeeth*, [History of Iraqi Medicine Pioneers], 32.

7. Interview by the author with Yousif 'Aqrawi in London, on December 12, 2005.

8. The higher number of Jewish students in the first years of the medical college was mainly due to the fact of their multilingual schooling at the Alliance Israelite, the famous Jewish school in Baghdad. There, in addition to English, students were taught Arabic and French. The school had a good reputation among Baghdad's educated elites. Muslim and Christian children were also sent to study at the school because it had higher standards than the Ottomans' state-run primary and secondary schools. For the history of the Jewish communities in modern Iraq, see Bashkin, *New Babylonians*.

9. Al-Witri and Shabandar, *Tareekh al-Tibb Fi al-'Iraq* [History of Medicine in Iraq].

10. The University of Al al-Bayt was inaugurated in 1924—three years before the establishment of the Royal College.

11. The word *Al al-Bayt* referred to the descendants of the house of the prophet Mohammed, a group revered by both Sunni and Shi'a Muslims. In addition to Islamic jurisprudence, the university was also meant to offer classes in an array of other fields, including the arts, law, engineering, and education. The Royal College was seen as an extension of this nationalizing project, which would be a crucible for Iraqi citizenship.

12. Under Ottoman rule, most Sunni education was provided through the Ottoman public school system, while Shi'a education was provided through independent Ja'fariyeh schools, run by the Shi'a clergy of the Hawza. As noted previously, Jewish students received their education from Baghdad and Basra branches of the Alliance Israelite, while many Christian students attended Jesuit schools. Al-Husri, *Muthakarati Fi al-'Iraq* [My Memoirs in Iraq], 420.

13. The problems surfaced in the clashes between Sati' al-Husri and Fahmi al-Mudarris, the general-director of the university.

14. The obstacles facing the foundation of the first Iraqi university were not merely due to local politics. This was also emphasized by international experts after a 1932 visit from the International Education Institute (IEI) to Iraq, headed by the famous American educator Paul Monroe. The IEI visited schools in different cities in Iraq and later hosted a conference on national higher education in the country's capital. The report written by Monroe concluded that establishing a university in Iraq was hasty and recommended the state continue to slowly expand colleges in different fields before attempting to assemble them all under the same administrative body of a university. Accompanying Monroe and contributing to the report was Monroe's Iraqi student Fadhil al-Jamali, son of a Shi'a cleric who served in different Iraqi government posts, including prime minister in 1953. For more details, see Monroe and Government of Iraq, *Report of the Educational Inquiry Commission*.

15. To this day, decades after the college was fully staffed by an all-Iraqi Arabic-speaking faculty, the council chooses English as the language of instruction. See al-Samara'i, *Hadeeth al-Thamaneen* [A Conversation at Eighty], Volume 4.

16. Private and public sector contributors included the Iranian Bank, Iraqi Petrol Company, Bank of the Orient, Ottoman Bank, Anglo-Persian Oil Company, Iraqi

Persian Company, and Andrew Weir Shipping Company. See al-Witri and Shabandar, *Tareekh al-Tibb Fi al-'Iraq*.

17. Ibid.

18. Al-Samara'i, *Hadeeth al-Thamaneen*, Volume 1, 154.

19. Ibid., 155–156.

20. The connections between body snatching and the rise of nineteenth-century Western medical education is well documented in scholarship. See Marshall, *Murdering to Dissect*; McCracken-Flesher, *The Doctor Dissected*; Hooper and Gormley, *Bodies for Sale*; Shultz, *Body Snatching*.

21. Sinderson, *Ten Thousand and One Nights*, 105.

22. Ibid.

23. Al-Witri and Shabandar, *Tareekh al-Tibb Fi al-'Iraq*, 104–105.

24. Ibid., 112.

25. Al-Samara'i, *Hadeeth al-Thamaneen*, Volume 1, 154.

26. Ibid., 154.

27. Many other Iraqi doctors who have written autobiographies from that period emphasize the importance of the formative years of the college in shaping their life trajectories and modes of being. Praises for the high standards and rigorous education that the unique experience of studying under British faculty offered prevailed in all these accounts.

28. Al-Samara'i, *Hadeeth al-Thamaneen*, Volume 1, 122–123.

29. Ibid., 124.

30. At the time of writing this chapter, the book had not been translated to the English language. Most of the translations are my own. Since then, there has been an official English translation of the memoir; see Zaki, *Memoir of an Iraqi Woman Doctor*.

31. Iraqi schools are divided into both science and literary curricula. Students usually choose to go to one or the other at a certain stage of their intermediate education. The science curriculum is much more in demand and, in many cases, the ranks of the literary program are filled by those rejected from the science curriculum.

32. Zaki, *Thikrayat Tabiba 'Iraqiyyah* [*Memoir of an Iraqi Woman Doctor*], 249.

33. Ibid.

34. Al-Witri, *Health Services in Iraq*.

35. Al-Witri's numbers are based on an Iraqi population estimated at around 5.5 million persons.

36. The first Minister of Social Affairs was Sami Shawkat, a well-known political figure and a medical doctor who returned to Iraq after World War I, having finished his training in Istanbul.

37. Sinderson, *Ten Thousand and One Nights*, 202.

38. Iraq was divided into fourteen *liwa*'s. The *liwa*' was further divided to *qadha*'s, which were in turn divided into *nahiya*s. If there were no adequate candidates from a particular *liwa*', candidates from a neighboring *liwa*' were to be selected.

39. Al-Witri, *Health Services in Iraq*, 7.

40. Sinderson, *Ten Thousand and One Nights*, 202.

41. Ibid.

42. Al-Witri, *Health Services in Iraq*, 8.

Chapter 5

1. Ferguson, "The Anti-Politics Machine: 'Development' and Bureaucratic Power in Lesotho," 180.

2. Critchley, "The Health of the Industrial Worker in Iraq," 73.

3. Salter, *Development of Iraq*.

4. Gran, *Beyond Eurocentrism*.

5. Al-Wardi, *Understanding Iraq*; Allawi, *The Occupation of Iraq*; al-Wardi, *Lamahat 'Ijtima'iyah Min Tareekh al-'Iraq al-Hadeeth*; al-Wardi, *Dirasah Fi Tabi'at al-Mujtama' al-'Iraqi*.

6. Al-Wardi, *Shakhsiyat al-Fard al-'Iraqi*.

7. Ibid., 44–45.

8. Al-Wardi's writings and proposals have had a wide reach among many educated Iraqis and have cultivated a range of debates and critiques in academic writings in Iraq and the Arabic-speaking world. See the special issue on Ali al-Wardi edited by Omar Dewachi in *Idafat*, Vols. 17 and 18, 2012.

9. In 2013, the US Naval Institute and the US army military journal, *Armor*, published the first major English translation of a collection of essays by al-Wardi. This translation was intended for both a general audience and a military audience. One of the most telling anecdotes in the book relays a conversation between a learned "counter-insurgent" detainee and his US military interrogator, where the detainee asserts that the US invasion is bound to fail due to the fact that the military had not read the work of al-Wardi and was therefore unfamiliar with Iraq's history and society. See Aboul-Enein, *Iraq in Turmoil*.

10. Anthropologists have shown and debated how such framings of "dual organization" exist and should not be seen as a hindrance to the understanding of ambivalence of the social order. See the famous essay by Claude Lévi-Strauss on the subject: *Structural Anthropology*, 132–166.

11. In her study *The Will to Improve* on development practices in Indonesia, Tania Murray Li makes a similar point about the internal contradictions that are imbued in such development projects that aimed at its parasitic relationship to its shortcomings and failures.

12. On the transformations in the social and political classes in Iraq, see Batatu, *The Old Social Classes and the Revolutionary Movements of Iraq*.

13. Salucci, *A People's History of Iraq*.

14. See Pieri, *Baghdad Arts Deco*, regarding the Minoprio and Doxiadis master plans of the city of Baghdad.

15. Salter, *Development of Iraq*.

16. There has been an abundance of literature on the history of the *'iqta'* in the south of Iraq, as well as on the Ottoman, British, and monarchy roles in defining and maintaining this tribal feudal system. See Haj, *The Making of Iraq, 1900–1963*; Batatu, *The Old Social Classes and the Revolutionary Movements of Iraq*; Cetinsaya, *The Ottoman Administration of Iraq, 1890–1908*; Tripp, *A History of Iraq*; Sluglett, *Britain in Iraq*; Abd al-Jabbar, *The Shi'ite Movement in Iraq*.

17. Many scholars have shown the consequences of development expertise and through their mobilization of technical and technocratic discourses have contributed to producing depoliticized narratives of society. Such discourses have played a central role in masking the political dimensions of development interventions, and both their intended and unintended consequences on social and economic life. See, for example, Ferguson, "The Anti-Politics Machine"; Li, *The Will to Improve*; Mitchell, *Rule of Experts*.

18. Salter, *Development of Iraq*, 2.

19. Fernea, "Land Reform and Ecology in Postrevolutionary Iraq," 358.

20. As others have shown, the role of the British was central in the amalgamation of social and economic powers of the *'iqta'* system—especially in the south of Iraq. See Batatu, *The Old Social Classes and the Revolutionary Movements of Iraq*; Fernea, *Shaykh and Effendi*; Haj, *The Making of Iraq, 1900–1963*.

21. Fisk, "Dujaila," 343.

22. Fernea continues, "This belief in the almost mystical efficacy of land ownership, transforming the tribal culture of the region into the Puritan culture of our own nineteenth century countryside, was shared by the Marxist reformists [of the 1958 revolution]." Fernea, "Land Reform and Ecology in Postrevolutionary Iraq," 357.

23. Ibid., 357–358.

24. A generation of Iraqi architects contributed to the expansion of the city through designing and implementing government buildings and structures. These architects developed unique concepts and techniques of mixing traditional and modern forms. These were the hope of the revival of Baghdad as a cosmopolitan city in tune with modern designs and appropriated traditional forms in the new designs of the city. See Chadirji, *Concepts and Influences*.

25. As urban historian Panayiota Plya argues, Doxiadis's modernist approach to post–World War II architecture avoided the political and imperial labeling of Western and socialist language. He emphasized "scientific legitimacy and cultural sensitivity" in his work, which he baptized as *Ekistics*, translated to the "science of human settlements." Doxiadis promised to incorporate the input of economics, geography, sociology, and anthropology, among other human sciences, which he "hoped would guard against designers' arbitrary self-expression and reconceptualize architecture and planning as rational processes of accommodating human needs." See Pyla, "Back to the Future: Doxiadis's Plans for Baghdad," 6.

26. According to Pyla, "[T]he core of Dynapolis was to expand continually along an axis to avert congestion, and the business district would grow along this axis controlled by zoning and the siting of public buildings, road systems, and green areas. The residential areas would also expand continually, along the core's flanks, echoing the open-ended logic of 'linear city' concepts, tracing back to Arturo Soria y Mata's 1882 Ciudad Lineal near Madrid and to Tony Garnier's Cite Industrielle (1901), not to mention the Soviet Linear Cities in the 1930s." Ibid., 8.

27. Ibid., 13.

28. *Sarayif*, plural of *sarifa*.

29. Other smaller settlements across Baghdad were more diverse and home to dwellers originating from other parts of the country, including the north.

30. Phillips, "Rural-to-Urban Migration in Iraq."

31. Ibid.

32. The marshes have been the center of attention of many travel writers and anthropologists both past and present, for their unique ecology and modes of life, which are often linked to the Sumarian civilization. See, for example, Eigeland, *When All the Lands Were Sea*; Field and Martin, *The Anthropology of Iraq*; Maxwell, *A Reed Shaken by the Wind*; Thesiger, *The Marsh Arabs*.

33. Al-Wardi, *Lamahat 'Ijtima'iyah Min Tareekh al-'Iraq al-Hadeeth*; Abd al-Jabbar and Dawod, *Tribes and Power*.

34. Al-Wardi, *Lamahat 'Ijtima'iyah Min Tareekh al-'Iraq al-Hadeeth*; al-Wardi, *Shakhsiyat al-Fard al-'Iraqi*.

35. During the 1940s and 1950s, the party led numerous nationwide demonstrations and workers' strikes criticizing the imperial policies of the pro-British government. The government cracked down on these demonstrations with the mobilization of the police and military, killing hundreds and imprisoning thousands of supporters. See Batatu, *The Old Social Classes and the Revolutionary Movements of Iraq*; Haj, *The Making of Iraq, 1900–1963*; Salucci, *A People's History of Iraq*.

36. Phillips, "Rural-to-Urban Migration in Iraq," 412.

37. Ibid., 412.

38. Ibid., 412.

39. Ibid., 421.

40. Ibid., 420.

41. The Baghdad Pact was a military alliance signed in 1955 between the UK government and the governments of Iraq, Turkey, Pakistan, and Iran, aiming to deter communist and Nasserist infiltration in the region.

42. Phillips, "Rural-to-Urban Migration in Iraq," 420.

43. The law also abolished the Tribal Disputes Codes—institutionalized by the British in rural Iraq after the end of World War I.

44. Haj, *The Making of Iraq, 1900–1963*, 121.

45. See the discussion of politics of the communist party and its relationship to the rationalization of the land reform in Haj, *The Making of Iraq, 1900–1963*.

46. Fernea, "Land Reform and Ecology in Postrevolutionary Iraq," 358.

47. Ibid., 359.

48. Pyla, "Back to the Future: Doxiadis's Plans for Baghdad."

49. Al-'Alousi, *Nostos*.

50. After the 2003 invasion and occupation, the city was once again renamed as Sadr City, celebrating the cleric Mohammed Baqir al-Sadr—the father of Moqtada al-Sadr, the leader of Shi'a Sadrist group—who was allegedly executed by the Saddam regime.

51. Phillips, "Rural-to-Urban Migration in Iraq," 420.

Chapter 6

1. Sayegh, *Child Survival in Wartime*, 1.

2. Alahmad and Keshavarzian, "A War on Multiple Fronts."

3. Up until recently, there has been little work documenting Iraqis' experiences of the Iran–Iraq war and its broader social significance. At that time, Iraq was closed to foreign research, and most of the writings from within the country were under strict censorship and monitoring by state security and colored by state war propaganda. Academic discourse about that period has been mostly concerned with the broader economic fallout and the Ba'th regime's consolidation of political power and repressive security apparatus. More recent work has also suggested that the Ba'th Party's wartime bureaucracy further cultivated a culture of militarization through its efforts to manage the country's war populations of soldiers, deserters, and martyrs' families. See Khoury, *Iraq in Wartime*.

4. As others have shown, Qasim's national plans were shaped by local concerns and more universal strategies evinced in other Eastern-bloc regimes. Such changes were more in tune with population strategies of other socialist health-care regimes of the time. See Batatu, *The Old Social Classes and the Revolutionary Movements of Iraq*; Haj, *The Making of Iraq, 1900–1963*; Salucci, *A People's History of Iraq*.

5. Ministry of Guidance, "Health under the Republican Regime."

6. Ibid.

7. In Iraq, most of state planning is defined in terms of the administrative mapping of the country. These are defined by the administrative units of governorate, the largest being Qada and the smallest being Nahiya. By 1965, this program had expanded and consisted of 171 centers located in the different *nahiyas*. These oversaw the work of 681 smaller centers in *baldaat*, which in turn were connected to 684 stand-alone dispensaries in the *qura*. See al-'Alwachi, *Tareekh al-Tib al-'Iraqi* [History of Iraqi Medicine].

8. These were based on the census of 1957, which was conducted during the monarchy.

9. Zakarian, "Organization and Conduction of Mass Smallpox Vaccination in Iraq with the Aid of the Soviet Union."

10. See al-'Alwachi, *Tareekh al-Tib al-'Iraqi*.

11. Interviews with senior Iraqi physicians.

12. Alnasrawi, *The Economy of Iraq*.

13. See Haba, *Formative Years of Computing in Iraq*, for a historical account of the development of electronic computing in Iraq during the sixties and seventies of the twentieth century, written by Iraqi pioneers and experts of computer science and engineering technology.

14. Personal communications and interviews with Iraqi government employees.

15. Alnasrawi, *The Economy of Iraq*, 102.

16. Alnasrawi, *The Economy of Iraq*.

17. As a result of the swelling of the military, Iraqi cities witnessed the proliferation of war attire with colors ranging from light khaki to dark-olive green. These differentiated soldier from officer, from party official, from popular army recruit.

18. Sayegh, *Child Survival in Wartime*.

19. Ibid.

20. Interview with Iraqi doctors in London.

21. Interview with Iraqi doctors.

22. Sell, "Egyptian International Labor Migration and Social Processes."

23. In 1989, after the end of the war and the demobilization of the Iraqi military, tens of thousands of Egyptian workers fled the country, going back to Egypt after being subjected to systematic harassment and abuse by their employers and government institutions. See some news coverage from the time: Cowell, "Egyptian Laborers Are Fleeing Iraq—*New York Times*." The majority of the remaining workers eventually left after the invasion of Kuwait in 1990. See also Fergany, "Aspects of Labor Migration and Unemployment in the Arab Region."

24. Efrati, "Productive or Reproductive? The Roles of Iraqi Women during the Iraq-Iran War"; Efrati, *Women in Iraq*.

25. One of Qasim's post-1958 interventions aimed to reform the personal status code with an attempt to give more equality to Iraqi women. He proposed outlawing polygamy and raising the minimum age of marriage to eighteen years. He also proposed that women would receive an equal share in inheritance—counter to common practices of family inherence that are based on Shari'a. Although Qasim's proposals were never implemented, they set in motion a new era of social reform that continued beyond the end of his rule. By the 1980s, Iraq had one of the highest rates of women's education in the Arab region. The progressive attitude toward women's education and economic independence during the republican era continued under Ba'th Party rule. In the 1970s, anthropologist Suad Joseph observed that the Ba'th framed women's employment not just as a means for national development, but also for the achievement of economic independence and the liberation of women themselves. See Joseph, "The Mobilization of Iraqi Women into the Wage Labor Force"; Joseph, "Elite Strategies for State-Building."

26. Jawaheri, *Women in Iraq*.

27. "Declaration of Alma-Ata, 1978."

28. Walsh and Warren, "Selective Primary Health Care."

29. Basilico et al., "Health for All? Competing Theories and Geopolitics."

30. Jolly, *Jim Grant*, 89.

31. Basilico et al., "Health for All? Competing Theories and Geopolitics."

32. The encouragement of reproduction resonated with the broader cultural values about marriage and fertility in Iraq and the broader Middle East. In other states in the Arab world, family planning and population control policies were enforced and were met with resistance and suspicion. See Inhorn, *Infertility and Patriarchy*; Inhorn, *Quest for Conception*; Ali, *Planning the Family in Egypt*.

33. Al-Ali, "Reconstructing Gender."

34. Sayegh, *Child Survival in Wartime*.

35. See Joseph, "The Mobilization of Iraqi Women into the Wage Labor Force"; Efrati, "Productive or Reproductive?"; Efrati, *Women in Iraq*; al-Ali, *Iraqi Women: Untold Stories from 1948 to the Present*; al-Ali, "Reconstructing Gender"; Neshat, "A Look into the Women's Movement in Iraq."

36. Scholars have shown the important role of this organization in pursuing women's rights and gender equality in Iraq during the 1970s and 1980s, despite tensions with the mainstream Ba'th Party leadership. See al-Ali, *Iraqi Women*; Efrati, "Productive or Reproductive? The Roles of Iraqi Women during the Iraq–Iran War"; al-Ali, "Reconstructing Gender"; Efrati, *Women in Iraq*.

37. Sayegh, *Child Survival in Wartime*, 25.

38. Ibid., 22.

39. Ibid., 22.

40. Ibid.

41. Ibid.

42. Ibid.

43. This increase in infant mortality is the most retrogressive infant-mortality statistic in the world—even in comparison with trends in sub-Saharan Africa, where the AIDS epidemic has taken a heavy toll on children. A study in 2005 reported that the mortality rate for children younger than five in Iraq years was 125 per 1,000 live births. This ratio is higher than all of Iraq's neighboring countries and far higher than before the US-led invasion, when that rate was 102 per 1,000 live births in 2002. See EMRO, WHO, "Iraq Family Health Survey Report."

Chapter 7

1. Hobsbawm, *The Age of Extremes*, 12.

2. The term *overseas doctor* has been commonly used in Britain to refer to doctors coming from outside the United Kingdom. In particular, it refers to the large population of doctors from India, Pakistan, and other former British colonies and commonwealth

countries. The term has been used less in British medical circles and has been replaced by the more politically correct term *international medical graduates* (IMG).

3. There is little information about the number of Asian doctors in Britain in the immediate establishment of the NHS in 1948. According to one account, there were close to 3,000 Asian doctors working in the NHS during the 1950s; see Esmail, "Asian Doctors in the NHS: Service and Betrayal." During the 1960s, close to 18,000 Asian doctors were employed by the NHS; see BBC, "How Asian Doctors Saved the NHS."

4. Only a quarter of each year's inflow of doctors to Britain, which ranged between 1,500 and 2,000 medical professionals, succeeded in acquiring full registration with the GMC.

5. According to Anwar and Ali, *Overseas Doctor*: "Generally the low status of overseas doctors in the NHS has been accompanied by poor training opportunities, thus forcing them into careers in the less attractive specialties," 7.

6. Several studies and reports emerged during this period to question the inherent discrimination against overseas doctors and their prospects for postgraduate training in the NHS. See Anwar and Ali, *Overseas Doctors*; Smith, *Overseas Doctors in the National Health Service*. Focusing on the precarious realities of overseas doctors in Britain, these accounts concluded that racial disadvantages were daily realities for these doctors. For more recent accounts discussing the history of that period and its consequences on the Asian doctor population in the United Kingdom, see Esmail, "Asian Doctors in the NHS: Service and Betrayal."

7. During the 1980s, the British right proposed the dismantling of what they deemed to be the "nanny state"—a depiction invoking the "overprotective" role of the welfare state and its interference in personal choice. They argued that the financial crisis and the long waiting lists of the NHS were mainly attributed to the overspending of the government and its inability to provide competitive, market-based services. As both purchaser and provider of health services, the NHS had no incentive to ensure a "good value for money" and failed to offer services that the consumers wanted in a timely fashion. See Sawer, "Gender, Metaphor and the State."

8. See Laurance, "Margaret Thatcher's Impact on the NHS." The trusts were public-sector corporations that were run by executive and non-executive boards and provided services on behalf of the NHS. "Health authorities ceased to run hospitals but instead 'purchased' care from hospitals."

9. The publication of the 1989 White Paper "Working for Patients" was significant. It became the blueprint of the restructuring of the institution vis-à-vis the new logics of state welfare. See HM Government, *Working for Patients*.

10. Woodyard, "Agenda: The Doctors' Malaise That Threatens Our Good Health/Shortage of NHS Doctors."

11. Ibid.

12. Casciani, "Overseas NHS Doctors 'Betrayed.'"

13. Fickling, "Foreign Doctors Rally against New Immigration Rules."

14. At the time of finishing this book (2016), the United Kingdom had just voted to leave the European Union (EU) in the historic "Brexit" vote. The consequences of this decision on the changing relationship between EU and overseas doctors are yet to become clear.

15. Casciani, "Overseas NHS Doctors 'Betrayed.'"

16. BBC, "Training the Refugee Doctors."

17. In the north of Iraq, the memory of the 1988 chemical attack on the village of Halabja was still fresh. Tens of thousands of Kurds from different cities and villages marched across the mountainous border with Turkey to seek a safe haven from the possibility of another chemical retaliation on the north. See Hiltermann, *A Poisonous Affair.*

18. In 1991, the UNHCR declared Iraq's refugee predicament a critical humanitarian crisis. Tens of thousands of Iraqis had become displaced in regional countries, claiming refugee status after the failed post-1991 Gulf War uprising that Saddam's regime viciously repressed. Escaping the retaliation for fear of reprisals, close to 33,000 people from southern Iraq crossed the border to Saudi Arabia, surrendering themselves to the US military and, in turn, were resettled in the nearby Saudi-run Rafha Refugee Camp. After enduring years of neglect and mistreatment—and after stories of Saudi camp guards' abuse of refugees leaked to the media—a total of 25,000 from the camp were swiftly resettled in the United States. See US Congress, "U.S. Committee for Refugees World Refugee Survey 1997—Saudi Arabia."

19. During the 1990s, Thailand had emerged as an international hub for the production of counterfeit passports. The Thai black market supplied high-quality documents for any nationality, for which they received a lot of media coverage. After 9/11, Western governments put a great deal of pressure on the Thai government to crack down on these black market networks, which extend from Bangkok to Canada. See Elias, "Man with 452 Passports: Brit Nabbed on Way to Scotland"; Fielding, "Going Cheap: The Fake Passports That Are Just a Phone Call Away"; Flanagan, "Briton Arrested in Thailand with 452 Forged Passports"; Goodell, "How to Fake a Passport"; Perry, "War on Terror Rise in Thefts and Forgeries as Fanatics Seek False Identities: Security Scare as Dvla 'Loses' 3,500 Passports"; Tang, "Thailand Emerges as Fake Passport Capital: Booming Trade in Forged Travel Documents Used by Criminal Underworld."

20. BBC, "1968: Race Discrimination Law Tightened."

21. Powell gained considerable support from the public, receiving more than 43,000 letters and 700 telegrams, which overloaded Wolverhampton's postal system. Only 4 telegrams and 800 letters expressed a form of hostility to him or his message.

22. Great Britain. Community Relations Commission, *Doctors from Overseas.*

23. Quoted in Anwar and Ali, *Overseas Doctors,* 10.

24. In 1975, S. K. Roy, an overseas Indian doctor working in Essex, wrote in the *British Medical Journal (BMJ)* criticizing not only the report but also questioning the function and role of the committee: "The Merrison Committee has acted as prosecutor,

jury, and judge of the overseas doctors, who now constitute 16% of general practitioners and 40% of junior hospital doctors in Britain. It is felt that the committee has given in to the pressure of groups who wish to restrict immigration of doctors for political reasons. It is well known that there has always been a vocal group who felt that their bargaining position was weakened by the presence of overseas doctors. See Roy, "Letter: Merrison Report and Overseas Doctors," 580.

25. See Chatterjee, "Letter: Test on Overseas Doctors"; Chatterjee, "Letter: Overseas Doctors in the Health Service"; Roy, "Letter: Merrison Report and Overseas Doctors."

26. Anwar and Ali, *Overseas Doctors*.

27. Leung, "Preparing for the PLAB Test," S163.

28. The two parts consist of 200 extended matching questions (EMQs) and single best answer (SBA) questions.

29. The test is administered in the following cities in India: Kolkata, Chennai, Mumbai, New Delhi, Hyderabad, and Bangalore.

30. Part Two is the objective structured clinical examination (OSCE), which represents about fourteen clinical scenarios or "stations." Each station is supervised by an examiner along with a "simulated patient." The latter is either an actor playing the role of a patient or a mannequin. The examinee is marked on his or her ability to "respect their privacy and dignity, and to attend to their comfort during the examination." Examinees need to perform a medical exam on the models as if they were real patients and must make sure that they do not "perform any actions on an anatomical model that would be unsafe or painful to a real person," which could even include "rectal or bimanual vaginal examination." See GMC, "At the PLAB Test."

31. Other communication skills include seeking informed consent or clarification for an invasive procedure, obtaining consent for a post-mortem, dealing with anxious patients or relatives, giving instructions on discharge, giving advice on lifestyle, promoting health, or communicating risk factors. See GMC, "At the PLAB Test."

32. One of the doctors who passed through Bridgend explained to me that the sudden surge in Iraqis in this small town raised some suspicion from the local ESL teacher and the local driving instructor.

33. Webster, *The National Health Service*, 1.

Conclusion

1. See for example Hansen and Stepputat, *States of Imagination*; Das and Poole, *Anthropology in the Margins of the State*; Nagengast, "Violence, Terror, and the Crisis of the State"; Gupta, *The Anthropology of the State*.

2. Das and Poole, *Anthropology in the Margins of the State*, 5.

3. Dewachi, "When Wounds Travel."

4. Essa et al., "Cancer Mortality in Basrah."

5. See Livingston, *Improvising Medicine: An African Oncology Ward in an Emerging Cancer Epidemic.*

6. See for example Dewachi, "The Toxicity of Everyday Survival in Iraq"; Gordts, "Iraq War Anniversary: Birth Defects and Cancer Rates at Devastating High in Basra and Fallujah"; Jamail, "Iraq: War's Legacy of Cancer."

7. Alaani et al., "Uranium and Other Contaminants in Hair from the Parents of Children with Congenital Anomalies in Fallujah, Iraq"; Busby, Hamdan, and Ariabi, "Cancer, Infant Mortality and Birth Sex-Ratio in Fallujah, Iraq 2005–2009."

8. Quoted in Jamail, "Iraq: War's Legacy of Cancer."

9. Ahmed, "How the World Health Organisation Covered up Iraq's Nuclear Nightmare"; Shah, "Iraqi Birth Defects Covered Up?"

10. Hickman and Ventura, *The Burn Pits.*

11. Calhoun, Murray, and Manring, "Multidrug-Resistant Organisms in Military Wounds from Iraq and Afghanistan."

12. Howard et al., "Acinetobacter Baumannii."

13. Petersen et al., "Trauma-Related Infections in Battlefield Casualties from Iraq."

14. Howard et al., "Acinetobacter Baumannii."

15. Necati Hakyemez et al., "Nosocomial Acinetobacter Baumannii Infections and Changing Antibiotic Resistance."

16. Grady, "Troops in Iraq Bring Resistant Bacteria Home."

17. To date, there have been only a handful of reports published by humanitarian hospitals (MSF and ICRC) that have indicated the higher rates of such organisms in war-related injuries treated by these organizations or their widespread incidence as a nosocomial infection. See for example Murphy et al., "Multidrug-Resistant Chronic Osteomyelitis Complicating War Injury in Iraqi Civilians."

Bibliography

Abd al-Jabbar, Faleh. *The Shi'ite Movement in Iraq*. London: Saqi, 2003.

Abd al-Jabbar, Faleh, and Hosham Dawod. *Tribes and Power: Nationalism and Ethnicity in the Middle East*. London: Saqi, 2001.

Abélès, Marc. *The Politics of Survival*. Translated by Julie Kleinman. Durham, NC: Duke University Press, 2009.

Aboul-Enein, Youssef H. *Iraq in Turmoil: Historical Perspectives of Dr. Ali Al-Wardi, From the Ottoman Empire to King Feisal*. Annapolis, MD: Naval Institute Press, 2012.

Adams, Vincanne. *Doctors for Democracy: Health Professionals in the Nepal Revolution*. Cambridge Studies in Medical Anthropology. Cambridge, England: Cambridge University Press, 1998.

Adorno, Theodor W., and Max Horkheimer. *Dialectic of Enlightenment*. London and New York: Verso, 1997.

Ahmed, Nafeez. "How the World Health Organisation Covered Up Iraq's Nuclear Nightmare." *The Guardian*, October 13, 2013. http://www.theguardian.com /environment/earth-insight/2013/oct/13/world-health-organisation-iraq-war -depleted-uranium.

Ahram, Ariel I. "Iraq in the Social Sciences: Testing the Limits of Research." *The Journal of the Middle East and Africa* 4.3 (October 1, 2013): 251–266.

Alaani, Samira, Muhammed Tafash, Christopher Busby, Malak Hamdan, and Eleonore Blaurock-Busch. "Uranium and Other Contaminants in Hair from the Parents of Children with Congenital Anomalies in Fallujah, Iraq." *Conflict and Health* 5 (September 2, 2011): 15.

Alahmad, Nida, and Arang Keshavarzian. "A War on Multiple Fronts." *Middle East Research and Information Report*, 257 (Winter 2010).

al-Ali, Nadje. "Reconstructing Gender: Iraqi Women between Dictatorship, War, Sanctions and Occupation." *Third World Quarterly* 26.4–5 (2005): 739–758.

———. *Iraqi Women: Untold Stories from 1948 to the Present*. London and New York: Zed Books, 2007.

al-'Alousi, Ma'ath. *Nostos: Hikayat Shari' Fi Baghdad* [Nostos: A Tale of a Street in Baghdad]. Beirut, Lebanon: Dar al-Furat, 2012.

al-'Alwachi, Abd al-Hamid. *Tareekh al-Tib al-'Iraqi* [History of Iraqi Medicine]. Baghdad: Matba'at al-As'ad, 1967.

al-Auwsi, Kawkeb. "Iraq's Doctors Are Subject to Humiliation and Murder." *Global Research,* 2013. http://www.globalresearch.ca/iraqs-doctors-are-subject-to -humiliation-and-murder/5343214.

al-Damalouji, Salim. *al-Kuliyyah al-Tibiyyah al-Malakiyyah al-'Iraqiyah: Min Khilal Seerah Thatiyah* [History of the Iraqi Royal College of Medicine through Autobiography]. Vol. 1. Beirut: al-Mu'assasah al-'Arabiyah Lildirasat Wa al-Nashir, 2003.

al-Husri, Sati'. *Muthakarati Fi al-'Iraq* [My Memoirs in Iraq]. Beirut: Dar al-Talee'a, 1967.

Ali, Kamran Asdar. *Planning the Family in Egypt: New Bodies, New Selves.* Modern Middle East series, 21. Austin, TX: University of Texas Press, 2002.

al-Kindi, Sadeer. "Violence against Doctors in Iraq." *The Lancet* 384.7 (September 2014): 954–955.

Allawi, Ali A. *The Occupation of Iraq: Winning the War, Losing the Peace.* New Haven, CT and London: Yale University Press, 2007.

———. *Faisal I of Iraq.* New Haven, CT and London: Yale University Press, 2014.

al-Mohammad, Hayder. "Ordure and Disorder: The Case of Basra and the Anthropology of Excrement." *Anthropology of the Middle East* 2.2 (September 30, 2007): 1–23.

———. "Relying on One's Tribe: A Snippet of Life in Basra Since the 2003 Invasion." *Anthropology Today* 26.6 (December 1, 2010): 23–26.

———. "Towards an Ethics of Being-With: Intertwinements of Life in Post-Invasion Basra." *Ethnos* 75, no. 4 (December 1, 2010): 425–46.

———. "'You Have Car Insurance, We Have Tribes': Negotiating Everyday Life in Basra and the Re-Emergence of Tribalism." *Anthropology of the Middle East* 6.1 (January 1, 2011): 18.

———. "A Kidnapping in Basra: The Struggles and Precariousness of Life in Post-Invasion Iraq." *Cultural Anthropology* 27.4 (November 2, 2012): 597–614.

al-Mohammad, Hayder, and Daniela Peluso. "Ethics and The 'Rough Ground' of the Everyday." *HAU: Journal of Ethnographic Theory* 2.2 (December 20, 2012): 42.

Alnasrawi, Abbas. *The Economy of Iraq: Oil, Wars, Destruction of Development and Prospects, 1950–2010.* Westport, CT: Greenwood Press, 1994.

al-Samara'i, Kamal. *Hadeeth al-Thamaneen: Seera Wa Thikrayat* [A Conversation at Eighty: A Biography and Memoir]. Vol. 1. Baghdad: Dar al-Shu'oun al-Thaqafiyyah al-'Ammah ('Afaq 'Arabyyah), 1994.

———. *Hadeeth al-Thamaneen: Seera Wa Thikrayat* [A Conversation at Eighty: A Biography and Memoir]. Vol. 4. Baghdad: Dar al-Shu'oun al-Thaqafiyyah al-'Ammah ('Afaq 'Arabyyah), 1997.

al-Wardi, Ali. *Dirasah Fi Tabi'at al-Mujtama' al-'Iraqi* [A Study in the Nature of Iraqi Society]. Baghdad: Maktabat al-'Ani, 1966.

————. *Lamahat 'Ijtima'iyah Min Tareekh al-'Iraq al-Hadeeth* [Social Glimpses of Modern Iraqi History]. London: Dar Kufaan, 1991.

————. *Understanding Iraq: Society, Culture, and Personality.* Lewiston, NY: Edwin Mellen, 2008.

————. *Shakhsiyat al-Fard al-'Iraqi* [The Nature of the Iraqi Personality]. Amman, Jordan: Dar al-Warraq, 2009.

al-Witri, Hashim. *Health Services in Iraq.* Vol. 2. Facts and Prospects in Iraq series. Baghdad: Iraqi Government Press, 1944.

al-Witri, Hashim, and Mu'ammar Shabandar. *Tareekh al-Tib Fi al-'Iraq* [History of Medicine in Iraq]. Baghdad: Iraqi Government Press, 1939.

Amar, Paul. *The Security Archipelago: Human-Security States, Sexuality Politics, and the End of Neoliberalism.* Durham, NC: Duke University Press, 2013.

Anderson, Warwick. *The Cultivation of Whiteness: Science, Health and Racial Destiny in Australia.* Carlton South, Australia: Melbourne University Press, 2002.

————. *Colonial Pathologies: American Tropical Medicine, Race, and Hygiene in the Philippines.* Durham, NC: Duke University Press, 2006.

————. "Making Global Health History: The Postcolonial Worldliness of Biomedicine." *Social History of Medicine.* 27.2 (2014): 372–384.

Anwar, Muhammad, and Ameer Ali. *Overseas Doctors: Experience and Expectations.* London: Commission for Racial Equality, 1987.

Arai, Masami. *Turkish Nationalism in the Young Turk Era.* Social, Economic, and Political Studies of the Middle East series. Leiden and New York: Brill, 1992.

Arnold, David. "Cholera and Colonialism in British India." *Past & Present* 113.1 (November 1, 1986): 118–151.

————. *Colonizing the Body: State Medicine and Epidemic Disease in Nineteenth-Century India.* Berkeley, CA: University of California Press, 1993.

————. *Warm Climates and Western Medicine: The Emergence of Tropical Medicine, 1500–1900.* Amsterdam and Atlanta: Rodopi, 1996.

————. "'Illusory Riches': Representations of the Tropical World, 1840–1950." *Singapore Journal of Tropical Geography* 21.1 (2000): 6–18.

Arrighi, Giovanni. "Hegemony Unravelling-1." *New Left Review* II.32 (April 2005): 23–80.

Ascherio, A., R. Chase, T. Coté, G. Dehaes, E. Hoskins, J. Laaouej, M. Passey, S. Qaderi, S. Shuqaidef, and M. C. Smith. "Effect of the Gulf War on Infant and Child Mortality in Iraq." *New England Journal of Medicine* 327.13 (September 24, 1992): 931–936.

Baghdadi, Abbas. *Baghdad Fi al-'Ishrinat* [Baghdad in the Twenties]. Beirut: al-Mu'assasah al-'Arabiyah Lildirasat Wa al-Nashir, 1999.

Bashkin, Orit. *New Babylonians: A History of Jews in Modern Iraq.* Stanford, CA: Stanford University Press, 2012.

Batatu, Hanna. *The Old Social Classes and the Revolutionary Movements of Iraq: A Study of Iraq's Old Landed and Commercial Classes and of Its Communists, Ba'thists and Free Officers*. Princeton, NJ: Princeton University Press, 1978.

BBC. "1968: Race Discrimination Law Tightened." *BBC*, November 26, 1968. http://news.bbc.co.uk/onthisday/hi/dates/stories/november/26/newsid_3220000/3220635.stm

———. "Training the Refugee Doctors." *BBC*, November 28, 2002. http://news.bbc.co.uk/2/hi/uk_news/2516797.stm

———. "How Asian Doctors Saved the NHS." *BBC*, November 26, 2003. http://news.bbc.co.uk/2/hi/health/3239540.stm.

———. "Iraqi Doctors to Be Allowed Guns." *BBC*, September 30, 2008. http://news.bbc.co.uk/2/hi/middle_east/7643766.stm

Bell, Heather. "Frontiers of Medicine in the Anglo-Egyptian Sudan, 1899–1940." Clarendon and Oxford, England: Oxford University Press, 1999.

Biehl, João. *Vita: Life in a Zone of Social Abandonment*, 1e. Berkeley, CA: University of California Press, 2005.

Biehl, João, and Adriana Petryna. *When People Come First: Critical Studies in Global Health*. Princeton, NJ: Princeton University Press, 2013.

Bouillon, Markus E. "Iraq's State-Building Enterprise: State Fragility, State Failure and a New Social Contract." *International Journal of Contemporary Iraqi Studies* 6.3 (September 1, 2012): 281–297.

Brotherton, P. Sean. *Revolutionary Medicine: Health and the Body in Post-Soviet Cuba*. Durham, NC: Duke University Press, 2012.

Burnham, Gilbert M., Riyadh Lafta, and Shannon Doocy. "Doctors Leaving 12 Tertiary Hospitals in Iraq, 2004–2007." *Social Science & Medicine* 69.2 (2009): 172–177.

Busby, Chris, Malak Hamdan, and Entesar Ariabi. "Cancer, Infant Mortality and Birth Sex-Ratio in Fallujah, Iraq 2005–2009." *International Journal of Environmental Research and Public Health* 7.7 (2010): 2828–2837.

Calhoun, Jason H., Clinton K. Murray, and M. M. Manring. "Multidrug-Resistant Organisms in Military Wounds from Iraq and Afghanistan." *Clinical Orthopaedics and Related Research* 466.6 (June 2008): 1356–1362.

"The Campaign in Iraq: A paper read before the Hunterian Society St George's Hospital on Feb 26th 1920." London: Wellcome Library. GC/93/1.

Casciani, Dominic. "Overseas NHS Doctors 'Betrayed.'" *BBC*, 2006. http://news.bbc.co.uk/2/hi/health/4928954.stm.

Cetinsaya, Gokhan. *The Ottoman Administration of Iraq, 1890–1908*, 1e. New York: Routledge, 2006.

Chadirji, Rifat. *Concepts and Influences: Towards a Regionalized International Architecture, 1952–1978*. Arlington, TX: KPI, 1986.

Chatterjee, S. S. "Letter: Overseas Doctors in the Health Service." *BMJ* 2.5966 (1975): 1085.

————. "Letter: Test on Overseas Doctors." *BMJ* 4.5995 (1975): 706.

Chesney, Francis Rawdon. "Reports on the Navigation of the Euphrates. Submitted to Government by Captain Chesney, Etc." Originally published in London: George Taylor, 1833. n.d.

————. *The Expedition for the Survey of the Rivers Euphrates and Tigris, Carried on by Order of the British Government in the Years 1835, 1836, and 1837; Preceded by Geographical and Historical Notices of the Regions Situated between the Rivers Nile and Indus.* London: Longman, Brown, Green, and Longmans, 1850.

————. *Narrative of the Euphrates Expedition Carried on by Order of the British Government during the Years 1835, 1836 and 1837.* London: Longmans, Green, 1868.

Choy, Catherine Ceniza. *Empire of Care: Nursing and Migration in Filipino American History.* American Encounters/Global Interactions. Durham, NC: Duke University Press, 2003.

Collier, Stephen J. *Post-Soviet Social: Neoliberalism, Social Modernity, Biopolitics.* Princeton, NJ: Princeton University Press, 2011.

Comaroff, Jean. "The Diseased Heart of Africa: Medicine, Colonialism, and the Black Body." In *Knowledge, Power, and Practice: The Anthopology of Medicine and Everyday Life*, eds. Shirley Lindenbaum and Margaret M. Lock. Berkeley, CA: University of California Press, 1993.

Court, C. "Iraq Sanctions Lead to Half a Million Child Deaths." *BMJ* (Clinical Research Ed.) 311.7019 (December 9, 1995): 1523.

Cowell, Alan, "Egyptian Laborers Are Fleeing Iraq." *New York Times*, November 15, 1989. Accessed July 22, 2013. http://www.nytimes.com/1989/11/15/world /egyptian-laborers-are-fleeing-iraq.html.

Critchley, A. Michael. "The Health of the Industrial Worker in Iraq." *British Journal of Industrial Medicine* 12.1 (January 1955): 73–75.

Das, Veena. *Critical Events: An Anthropological Perspective on Contemporary India.* Delhi and New York: Oxford University Press, 1995.

Das, Veena, and Deborah Poole. *Anthropology in the Margins of the State.* School of American Research Press, 2004.

Davis, Eric. *Memories of State: Politics, History, and Collective Identity in Modern Iraq,* 1e. Berkeley, CA: University of California Press, 2005.

"Declaration of Alma-Ata, 1978." World Health Organization. Accessed July 21, 2013. http://www.euro.who.int/en/who-we-are/policy-documents/declaration-of-alma -ata,-1978.

Dewachi, Omar. "Al-Wardi wa Geneologia al-Khitab al-Thaqafi [Al-Wardi and the Genealogy of Cultural Discourse]." *Idafat* 17–18 (2012): 4–8.

————. "The Toxicity of Everyday Survival in Iraq." *Jadaliyya*, August 13, 2013. http:// www.jadaliyya.com/pages/index/13537/the-toxicity-of-everyday-survival-in-iraq.

————. "When Wounds Travel." *Medicine Anthropology Theory* 2.2 (2015): 61–82.

Dewachi, Omar, Mac Skelton, Vinh-Kim Nguyen, Fouad M. Fouad, Ghassan Abu Sitta, Zeina Maasri, and Rita Giacaman. "Changing Therapeutic Geographies of the Iraqi and Syrian Wars." *The Lancet* 383.9915 (February 2014): 449–457.

Dodge, Toby. *Inventing Iraq: The Failure of Nation-Building and a History Denied.* New York: Columbia University Press, 2003.

Efrati, Noga. "Productive or Reproductive? The Roles of Iraqi Women during the Iraq-Iran War." *Middle Eastern Studies* 35.2 (April 1, 1999): 27–44.

———. *Women in Iraq: Past Meets Present.* New York: Columbia University Press, 2012.

Eigeland, Tor. *When All the Lands Were Sea: A Photographic Journey into the Lives of the Marsh Arabs of Iraq.* Northampton, MA: Olive Branch Press, 2014.

Elias, Richard. "Man with 452 Passports; Brit Nabbed on Way to Scotland." *Daily Record*, 2005.

Elshakry, Marwa. *Reading Darwin in Arabic, 1860–1950.* Chicago: University of Chicago Press, 2016.

EMRO, WHO. "Iraq Family Health Survey Report." EMRO, 2006. http://www.emro.who.int/iraq/.

Engelhardt, Édouard Philippe. *La Turquie et Le Tanzimât; Ou: Histoire Des Réformes Dans L'empire Ottoman Depuis 1826 Jusqu'à Nos Jours.* University of California Libraries, 1882.

Esmail, Aneez. "Asian Doctors in the NHS: Service and Betrayal." *The British Journal of General Practice* 57.543 (October 1, 2007): 827–834.

Essa, Sajjad S., Omran S. Habib, Jasim M. A. al-Diab, Kareem A. S. al-Imara, and Narjis A. H. Ajeel. "Cancer Mortality in Basrah." *The Medical Journal of Basrah University* 25.1 (2007): 55–60.

Fahmy, Khaled. *All the Pasha's Men: Mehmed Ali, His Army and the Making of Modern Egypt.* Cairo: The American University in Cairo Press, 2010.

Farmer, Paul, Arthur Kleinman, Jim Kim, and Matthew Basilico. *Reimagining Global Health: An Introduction.* Berkeley, CA: University of California Press, 2013.

Farouk-Sluglett, Marion, and Peter Sluglett. "The Historiography of Modern Iraq." *The American Historical Review* 96.5 (December 1, 1991): 1408–1421.

Fassin, Didier. "Another Politics of Life Is Possible." *Theory, Culture & Society* 26.5 (September 1, 2009): 44–60.

Fergany, Nader. "Aspects of Labor Migration and Unemployment in the Arab Region." Almishkat Center for Research, Cairo 3 (2001). http://www.mafhoum.com/press4/116S25.pdf.

Ferguson, James. "The Anti-Politics Machine: 'Development' and Bureaucratic Power in Lesotho." *The Ecologist* 24.5 (October 1994): 176–181.

Fernea, Robert A. "Land Reform and Ecology in Postrevolutionary Iraq." *Economic Development and Cultural Change* 17.3 (April 1, 1969): 356–381.

Fernea, Robert A. *Shaykh and Effendi: Changing Patterns of Authority among the El Shabana of Southern Iraq.* Cambridge, MA: Harvard University Press, 1970.

Fickling, David. "Foreign Doctors Rally against New Immigration Rules." *The Guardian*, 2006.

Field, Henry, and Richard C. Martin. *The Anthropology of Iraq*. Vols. 469, 631. Publication (Field Museum of Natural History). Chicago: Field Museum, 1940.

Fielding, Nick. "Going Cheap: The Fake Passports That Are Just a Phone Call Away." *Times Online*, 2004. http://www.timesonline.co.uk/tol/news/uk/article1033299.ece.

Fischer, Michael M. J. *Emergent Forms of Life and the Anthropological Voice*. Durham, NC: Duke University Press, 2003.

Fisk, Brad. "Dujaila: Iraq's Pilot Project for Land Settlement." *Economic Geography* 28.4 (October 1, 1952): 343–354.

Fkaiki, Adeeb Tawfeeq. *Tarikh a'lam al-Tibb al-'Iraqi al-Hadeeth* [History of Iraqi Medicine Pioneers]. Baghdad: Dar al-Hureyyah, 1989.

Flanagan, Padraic. "Briton Arrested in Thailand with 452 Forged Passports." *The Express*, 2005.

Fortna, Benjamin C. *Imperial Classroom: Islam, the State, and Education in the Late Ottoman Empire*. Oxford: Oxford University Press, 2002.

Foucault, Michel. *"Society Must Be Defended": Lectures at the Collège de France, 1975–1976*. London: Picador, 2003.

———. *Security, Territory, Population: Lectures at the Collège de France 1977–1978*. London: Picador, 2009.

———. "The Politics of Health in the Eighteenth Century." *Foucault Studies* 0.18 (October 17, 2014): 113–127.

Garfield, Richard. "Morbidity and Mortality Among Iraqi Children from 1990 Through 1998: Assessing the Impact of the Gulf War and Economic Sanctions." New York: Columbia University, 1999. http://www.casi.org.uk/info/garfield/dr-garfield.html.

GMC. "At the PLAB Test." Accessed May 25, 2014. http://www.gmc-uk.org/doctors/plab/advice_part2.asp#1.

Good, Mary-Jo DelVecchio. *American Medicine: The Quest for Competence*. Berkeley, CA: University of California Press, 1995.

Goodell, Jeff. "How to Fake a Passport." *New York Times*, 2002.

Gordon, Joy. "Economic Sanctions and Global Governance: The Case of Iraq." *Global Crime* 10.4 (October 22, 2009): 356–367.

———. *Invisible War: The United States and the Iraq Sanctions*. Cambridge, MA: Harvard University Press, 2012.

Gordts, Eline. "Iraq War Anniversary: Birth Defects and Cancer Rates at Devastating High in Basra and Fallujah." *Huffington Post*, 2013. http://www.huffingtonpost.com/2013/03/20/iraq-war-anniversary-birth-defects-cancer_n_2917701.html.

Government of 'Iraq. *Annual Report of the Health Department for the Years 1923–1924*. Baghdad: Government Press, Baghdad, 1925.

Grady, Denise. "Troops in Iraq Bring Resistant Bacteria Home." *New York Times*, August 4, 2005. http://www.nytimes.com/2005/08/04/us/troops-in-iraq-bring-resistant-bacteria-home.html.

Gran, Peter. *Beyond Eurocentrism: A New View of Modern World History*. Syracuse, NY: Syracuse University Press, 1996.

Great Britain. Foreign Office. Historical Section. "Mesopotamia: Handbook Prepared under the Direction of the Historical Section of the Foreign Office-No. 63." His Majesty's Stationery Office, 1920.

———. Colonial Office. "Report by His Majesty's Government on the Administration of 'Iraq for the Period April, 1923–December, 1924." London: His Majesty's Stationery Office, 1925.

———. Colonial Office. Special Report by His Majesty's Government in the United Kingdom of Great Britain and Northern Ireland to the Council of the League of Nations on the Progress of Iraq during the Period 1920–1931." No. 58. London: His Majesty's Stationery Office, 1931.

———. Community Relations Commission. Doctors from Overseas? A Case for Consultation. London: Reference and Community Services, Community Relations Commission, 1976.

Gupta, Akhil. *The Anthropology of the State: A Reader*, 1e. Malden, MA and Oxford: Wiley-Blackwell, 2005.

Haba, Zaid, ed. *Formative Years of Computing in Iraq*. CreateSpace Independent Publishing Platform, 2015.

Haddad, William W., and William Ochsenwald. *Nationalism in a Non-National State: The Dissolution of the Ottoman Empire*. Columbus, OH: Ohio State University Press, 1977.

Haffkine, W. M. "A Lecture: Preventive Inoculation Against Cholera in India." *The Lancet* 146.3773 (December 1895): 1555–1556.

Haj, Samira. *The Making of Iraq, 1900–1963: Capital, Power, and Ideology*. Social and Economic History of the Middle East SUNY series. Albany, NY: State University of New York Press, 1997.

Hall, S., and D. Olafimihan. "A Dose of the UN's Medicine." *Nursing Times* 94.24 (June 17, 1998): 12–13.

Hallinan, T. J. "Report of Inspector-General of Health Services, the Iraqi Health Services for the Years 1925 & 1926." Baghdad: Government Press, 1928.

Han, Clara. *Life in Debt: Times of Care and Violence in Neoliberal Chile*. Berkeley, CA: University of California Press, 2012.

Hanioğlu, M. Şükrü. *A Brief History of the Late Ottoman Empire*. Princeton, NJ: Princeton University Press, 2010.

Hansen, Thomas Blom, and Finn Stepputat. *States of Imagination: Ethnographic Explorations of the Postcolonial State*. Politics, History, and Culture series. Durham, NC: Duke University Press, 2001.

Harrison, Mark. *The Medical War: British Military Medicine in the First World War*. Oxford: Oxford University Press, 2010.

Headrick, Daniel R. *The Tools of Empire: Technology and European Imperialism in the Nineteenth Century*. New York: Oxford University Press, 1981.

Heffernan, Michael. "Geography, Cartography and Military Intelligence: The Royal Geographical Society and the First World War." *Transactions of the Institute of British Geographer* 21.3 (1996): 504–533.

Heggs, T. Barrett. "Annual Report of the Health Department for the Year 1921." Baghdad: Government Press, 1922.

Hickman, Joseph, and Jesse Ventura. *The Burn Pits: The Poisoning of America's Soldiers*. New York: Hot Books, 2016.

Higgins, Benjamin H. "World War I and Its Effects on British Financial Institutions." *Lombard Street in War and Reconstruction*, 10–25. NBER, 1949.

Hiltermann, Joost R. *A Poisonous Affair: America, Iraq, and the Gassing of Halabja*, 1e. Cambridge, England: Cambridge University Press, 2007.

HM Government. *Working for Patients*. London: The Stationary, 1989.

Hobsbawm, Eric. *The Age of Extremes: 1914–1991*. New edition. London and New York: Abacus, 1995.

Hooper, Mary, and Greg Gormley. *Bodies for Sale: A Tale of Victorian Tomb-Robbers*. New York and London: Franklin Watts, 1999.

Howard, Aoife, Michael O'Donoghue, Audrey Feeney, and Roy D. Sleator. "Acinetobacter Baumannii." *Virulence* 3.3 (May 1, 2012): 243–250. doi:10.4161/viru.19700.

Iliffe, John. *East African Doctors: A History of the Modern Profession*. African Studies series; 95. Cambridge and New York: Cambridge University Press, 1998.

Inda, Jonathan Xavier. *Anthropologies of Modernity: Foucault, Governmentality, and Life Politics*. Malden, MA: Blackwell, 2005.

"Infrastructure: Introductory Commentary by AbdouMaliq Simone—Cultural Anthropology." Accessed October 7, 2014. http://www.culanth.org/curated_collections /11-infrastructure/discussions/12-infrastructure-introductory-commentary-by -abdoumaliq-simone.

Inhorn, Marcia Claire. *Quest for Conception: Gender, Infertility, and Egyptian Medical Traditions*. Philadelphia, PA: University of Pennsylvania Press, 1994.

———. *Infertility and Patriarchy: The Cultural Politics of Gender and Family Life in Egypt*. Philadelphia: University of Pennsylvania Press, 1996.

"Inoculations Against Cholera in India." *British Medical Journal* 2.1812 (September 21, 1895): 735–739.

Isaacs, Haskell. "Britain's Contribution to Medicine and the Teaching of Medicine in Iraq." *Bulletin* (British Society for Middle Eastern Studies) 3.1 (1976): 20–28.

Jamail, Daher. "Iraq: War's Legacy of Cancer." News. Aljazeera, March 15, 2013. http://www.aljazeera.com/indepth/features/2013/03/2013315171951838638.html.

Jawaheri, Yasmin Husein. *Women in Iraq: The Gender Impact of International Sanctions*. London: Tauris, 2008.

Jolly, Richard. *Jim Grant: UNICEF Visionary*. Florence, Italy: UNICEF, 2001.

Jones, J. T. "Journal of a Steam Voyage to the North of Baghdad, in April, 1846." *Journal of the Royal Geographical Society of London* 18 (1848): 1–19.

Joseph, Suad. "Elite Strategies for State-Building: Women, Family, Religion and State in Iraq and Lebanon." *Women, Islam and the State*, ed. Deniz Kandiyoti. (Philadelphia, PA: Temple University Press), 176–200.

———. "The Mobilization of Iraqi Women into the Wage Labor Force." *Studies in Third World Societies* 16 (1982): 69–90.

Kâhya, Esin, and Aysegül Demirhan Erdemir. *Medicine in the Ottoman Empire: And Other Scientific Developments*. Istanbul: Nobel Medical Publications, 1997.

Kayali, Hasan. *Arabs and Young Turks: Ottomanism, Arabism, and Islamism in the Ottoman Empire, 1908–1918*. Berkeley, CA: University of California Press, 1997.

Keshavjee, Salmaan. *Blind Spot: How Neoliberalism Infiltrated Global Health*. Oakland, CA: University of California Press, 2014.

Khoury, Dina Rizk. "Iraq's Lost Cultural Heritage." *Perspectives on History*, September 2003. https://www.historians.org/publications-and-directories/perspectives-on -history/september-2003/iraqs-lost-cultural-heritage#.

———. *Iraq in Wartime: Soldiering, Martyrdom, and Remembrance*. Cambridge: Cambridge University Press, 2013.

Kim, Jim Yong, Joyce V. Millen, Alec Irwin, and John Gershman, eds. *Dying for Growth: Global Inequality and the Health of the Poor*, 1e. Monroe, ME: Common Courage Press, 2002.

Lane, W. B. "Administration Report of the Health Department 1919–1920." Baghdad: Government Press, 1921.

Larkin, Brian. "The Politics and Poetics of Infrastructure." *Annual Review of Anthropology* 42.1 (2013): 327–343.

Laurance, Jeremy. "Margaret Thatcher's Impact on the NHS." *The Independent*. Accessed May 25, 2014. http://www.independent.co.uk/news/uk/politics/margaret -thatchers-impact-on-the-nhs-8564758.html.

Lawrence, T. E. "T. E. Lawrence to Lord Curzon," September 27, 1919. F.O. No. 134231. http://www.telstudies.org/writings/letters/1919-20/190927_curzon.shtml.

Leader. "Ungoverned and Ungovernable." *The Guardian*, April 14, 2006. http://www .theguardian.com/commentisfree/2006/apr/14/iraq.comment.

Lemke, Thomas. *Biopolitics: An Advanced Introduction*, 1e. New York: New York University Press, 2011.

———. "Foucault, Politics, and Failure: A Critical Review of Studies of Governmentality." *Foucault, Biopolitics, and Governmentality*, eds. Jakob Nilsson and Sven-Olov Wallenstein, 35–52. Huddinge: Södertörn University, 2013.

———. *Foucault, Governmentality, and Critique*. New York: Routledge, 2015.

Leung, Wai-Ching. "Preparing for the PLAB Test." *BMJ Career Focus* 325.7373 (2002): S163.

Lévi-Strauss, Claude. *Structural Anthropology*. New York: Basic, 1963.

Li, Tania Murray. *The Will to Improve: Governmentality, Development, and the Practice of Politics*. Durham, NC: Duke University Press, 2007.

Linebagh, Peter. "May Day at Kut and Kenthal." *Counterpunch*, April 30, 2003. http://
www.counterpunch.org/2003/04/30/may-day-at-kut-and-kenthal/print.

Livingston, Julie. *Improvising Medicine: An African Oncology Ward in an Emerging Cancer Epidemic*. Durham, NC: Duke University Press, 2012.

Lock, Margaret, and Vinh-Kim Nguyen. *An Anthropology of Biomedicine*. New York: Wiley, 2010.

Lockrem, Jessica, and Adonia Lugo. "Infrastructure." *Cultural Anthropology*. Accessed December 12, 2016. https://culanth.org/curated_collections/11-infrastructure.

Loftus, William Kennett. "Notes of a Journey from Baghdad to Busrah, with Descriptions of Several Chaldaean Remains." *Journal of the Royal Geographical Society of London* 26 (1856): 131–153.

Lynch, Henry. "Note Accompanying a Survey of the Tigris between Ctesiphone and Mosul." *Journal of the Royal Geographical Society of London* 9 (1839): 441–442.

Ma'oz, Moshe. *Ottoman Reform in Syria and Palestine, 1840–1861: The Impact of the Tanzimat on Politics and Society*, 1e. Oxford: Oxford University Press, 1968.

Main, Ernest. *Iraq from Mandate to Independence*. London: Allen & Unwin, 1935.

Makiya, Kanan. *Republic of Fear: The Politics of Modern Iraq*. Berkeley, CA: University of California Press, 1998.

Marshall, Tim. *Murdering to Dissect: Graverobbing, Frankenstein, and the Anatomy Literature*, 1e. Manchester: Manchester University Press, 1996.

Matthew Basilico, Jonathan Weigel, Anjali Motgi, Jacob Bor, and Salmaan Keshavjee. "Health for All? Competing Theories and Geopolitics." *Reimagining Global Health*. Berkeley, CA: University of California Press, 2012.

Maude, Stanley. "The Proclamation of Baghdad." World War I Document Archive. Accessed December 13, 2016. https://wwi.lib.byu.edu/index.php/The_Proclamation _of_Baghdad.

Maxwell, Gavin. *A Reed Shaken by the Wind: Travels Among the Marsh Arabs of Iraq*. London: Eland, 2004.

Mbembe, Achille. *On the Postcolony*, 1e. Berkeley, CA: University of California Press, 2001.

———. "Necropolitics." *Public Culture* 15.1 (2003): 11–40.

McCracken-Flesher, Caroline. *The Doctor Dissected: A Cultural Autopsy of the Burke and Hare Murders*. Oxford: Oxford University Press, 2011.

Merton, Robert K. "The Unanticipated Consequences of Purposive Social Action." *American Sociological Review* 1.6 (1936): 894–904.

Mesopotamian Expeditionary Force. Mesopotamia Civil Medical Service. Baghdad L/PS/10/771, 1918a.

———. Preliminary Scheme of Civil Medical Provision for Mesopotamia. Baghdad L /PS/10/771, 1918b.

Ministry of Guidance. "Health under the Republican Regime." Baghdad: Government of Iraq Press, 1960.

Mitchell, Timothy. *Rule of Experts: Egypt, Techno-Politics, Modernity*. Berkeley, CA: University of California Press, 2002.

Monroe, Paul, and Government of Iraq, Educational Inquiry Commission. *Report of the Educational Inquiry Commission*. Government Press, 1932.

Montgomery, Bruce P. "Immortality in the Secret Police Files: The Iraq Memory Foundation and the Baath Party Archive." *International Journal of Cultural Property* 18.3 (August 2011): 309–336.

Morris, James. *Farewell the Trumpets: An Imperial Retreat*, 1e. New York: Mariner, 1980.

Moulin, Anne Marie. "Tropical without the Tropics: The Turning Point of Pasteurian Medicine in North Africa." *Warm Climates and Western Medicine: The Emergence of Tropical Medicine, 1500–1900*, ed. David Arnold, 160–180. The Wellcome Institute History of Medicine series. Amsterdam and Atlanta: Rodopi, 1996.

Murphy, Richard A., Jean-Baptiste Ronat, Rasheed M. Fakhri, Patrick Herard, Nikki Blackwell, Sophie Abgrall, and Deverick J. Anderson. "Multidrug-Resistant Chronic Osteomyelitis Complicating War Injury in Iraqi Civilians." *The Journal of Trauma* 71.1 (July 2011): 252–254.

Nagengast, Carole. "Violence, Terror, and the Crisis of the State." *Annual Review of Anthropology* 23.1 (1994): 109–136. doi:10.1146/annurev.an.23.100194.000545.

Necati Hakyemez, Ismail, Abdulkadir Kucukbayrak, Tekin Tas, Aslihan Burcu Yikilgan, Akcan Akkaya, Aliye Yasayacak, and Hayrettin Akdeniz. "Nosocomial Acinetobacter Baumannii Infections and Changing Antibiotic Resistance." *Pakistan Journal of Medical Sciences* 29.5 (2013): 1245–1248.

Neshat, Saeid N. "A Look into the Women's Movement in Iraq." *Farzaneh* 6.11 (2003): 54.

Nguyen, Vinh-Kim. *The Republic of Therapy: Triage and Sovereignty in West Africa's Time of AIDS*, 1e. Durham, NC: Duke University Press, 2010.

Omissi, David E. *Air Power and Colonial Control: The Royal Air Force 1919–1939*, 1e. Manchester and New York: Manchester University Press, 1990.

Ong, Aihwa, and Stephen J. Collier. *Global Assemblages: Technology, Politics, and Ethics as Anthropological Problems*. Malden, MA: Blackwell, 2005.

Paley, Amit R. "Iraqi Hospitals Are War's New 'Killing Fields.'" *The Washington Post*, August 30, 2006. http://www.washingtonpost.com/wp-dyn/content/article/2006/08/29/AR2006082901680.html.

Patel, Abdulrazzak. *The Arab Nahdah: The Making of the Intellectual and Humanist Movement*, 1e. Edinburgh, Scotland: Edinburgh University Press, 2013.

Perry, Keith. "War on Terror Rise in Thefts and Forgeries as Fanatics Seek False Identities: Security Scare as Dvla 'Loses' 3,500 Passports." *The Express*, 2002.

Petersen K., Riddle M. S., Danko J. R., et al. "Trauma-Related Infections in Battlefield Casualties from Iraq." *Annals of Surgery* 245.5 (2007): 803–811.

Petryna, Adriana. *When Experiments Travel: Clinical Trials and the Global Search for Human Subjects*, 1e. Princeton, NJ: Princeton University Press, 2009.

Phillips, Doris G. "Rural-to-Urban Migration in Iraq." *Economic Development and Cultural Change* 7.4 (July 1, 1959): 405–421.

Pick, Daniel. *Faces of Degeneration: A European Disorder*, c. 1848–1918. Cambridge: Cambridge University Press, 1993.

Pieri, Caecilia. *Baghdad Arts Deco: Architectural Brickwork, 1920–1950*. Cairo, Egypt; New York: The American University in Cairo Press, 2011.

Pormann, Peter. "The Arab 'Cultural Awakening (Nahda),' 1870–1950, and the Classical Tradition." *International Journal of the Classical Tradition* 13.1 (2006): 3–20.

Porter, Dorothy. *The History of Public Health and the Modern State*. Amsterdam: Rodopi, 1994.

———. *Health, Civilization, and the State: A History of Public Health from Ancient to Modern Times*. London and New York: Routledge, 1999.

———. "How Did Social Medicine Evolve, and Where Is It Heading?" *PLoS Med* 3.10 (October 24, 2006): e399. doi:10.1371/journal.pmed.0030399.

Povinelli, Elizabeth A. *Economies of Abandonment: Social Belonging and Endurance in Late Liberalism*. Durham, NC: Duke University Press, 2011.

Prince, Ruth J., and Rebecca Marsland. *Making and Unmaking Public Health in Africa: Ethnographic and Historical Perspectives*. Athens, OH: Ohio University Press, 2013.

Pyla, Panayiota. "Back to the Future: Doxiadis's Plans for Baghdad." *Journal of Planning History* 7.3 (2008): 3–19.

Pylypa, Jen. "Power and Bodily Practice: Applying the Work of Foucault to an Anthropology of the Body." *Arizona Anthropologist* 13.0 (1998): 21–36.

Quataert, Donald. *The Ottoman Empire, 1700–1922*. Cambridge: Cambridge University Press, 2005.

Rabinow, Paul. *French Modern: Norms and Forms of the Social Environment*. Chicago: University of Chicago Press, 1995.

Rabinow, Paul, and Nikolas Rose. "Biopower Today." *BioSocieties* 1.2 (June 19, 2006): 195–217.

Redfield, Peter. *Life in Crisis: The Ethical Journey of Doctors without Borders*. Berkeley, CA: University of California Press, 2013.

Reynolds, Paul. "Iraq the Ungovernable." *BBC*, August 20, 2003. http://news.bbc .co.uk/2/hi/middle_east/3166797.stm.

Rogan, Eugene. *The Fall of the Ottomans: The Great War in the Middle East*. New York: Basic, 2015.

Rogaski, Ruth. *Hygienic Modernity: Meanings of Health and Disease in Treaty-Port China*. Berkeley: University of California Press, 2004.

Rose, Nikolas. *The Politics of Life Itself: Biomedicine, Power, and Subjectivity in the Twenty-First Century*. Princeton, NJ: Princeton University Press, 2006.

Roy, S. K. "Letter: Merrison Report and Overseas Doctors." *BMJ* 4.5996 (1975): 579–580.

Said, Edward W. *Orientalism*. Vol. 1. New York: Vintage, 1979.

Saleh, Zaki. *Britain and Mesopotamia (Iraq to 1914): A Study in British Foreign Affairs.* Baghdad: al-Ma'arif, 1966.

Salter, James Arthur. *Development of Iraq: A Plan of Action.* London: Caxton, 1955.

Salucci, Ilario. *A People's History of Iraq: The Iraqi Communist Party, Workers' Movements and the Left 1924–2004.* Chicago: Haymarket, 2005.

Sassoon, Joseph. *Saddam Hussein's Ba'ath Party.* Cambridge: Cambridge University Press, 2011.

Sawer, Marian. "Gender, Metaphor and the State." *Feminist Review* 52 (1996): 118.

Sayegh, Juliette. *Child Survival in Wartime: A Case Study from Iraq 1983–1989.* The Department of Population Dynamics, The Johns Hopkins School of Hygiene and Public Health, 1992.

Scott, James C. *The Art of Not Being Governed: An Anarchist History of Upland Southeast Asia.* New Haven, CT: Yale University Press, 2010.

———. *Weapons of the Weak: Everyday Forms of Peasant Resistance.* New Haven, CT: Yale University Press, 1985.

Sell, Ralph R. "Egyptian International Labor Migration and Social Processes: Toward Regional Integration." *The International Migration Review* 22.3 (1988): 87–108.

Shah, Jeena. "Iraqi Birth Defects Covered Up?" *The Huffington Post*, January 4, 2013. http://www.huffingtonpost.com/the-center-for-constitutional-rights/iraqi-birth-defects-cover_b_4046442.html.

Shultz, Suzanne M. *Body Snatching: The Robbing of Graves for the Education of Physicians in Early Nineteenth Century America*, 1e. Jefferson, NC: McFarland, 2005.

Simon, Reeva S. *Iraq Between the Two World Wars: The Militarist Origins of Tyranny.* New York: Columbia University Press, 2004.

Simone, AbdouMaliq. "People as Infrastructure: Intersecting Fragments in Johannesburg." *Public Culture* 16.3 (September 21, 2004): 407–429.

Sinderson, Harry Chapman. "Some Recollections of Iraq, 1918–1946." *Med Press* 22.9 (1949): 221–224.

———. *Ten Thousand and One Nights: Memories of Iraq's Sherifian Dynasty.* London: Hodder & Stroughton, 1973.

Sluglett, Peter. *Britain in Iraq: Contriving King and Country, 1914–1932.* New York: Columbia University Press, 2007.

Smith, D. J. *Overseas Doctors in the National Health Service.* Oxford: Heinemann, 1980.

Stedman Jones, Gareth. *Outcast London: A Study in the Relationship between Classes in Victorian Society.* New York: Pantheon, 1984.

Stoler, Ann Laura. *Race and the Education of Desire: Foucault's History of Sexuality and the Colonial Order of Things.* Durham, NC and London: Duke University Press, 1995.

Tang, Alisa. "Thailand Emerges as Fake Passport Capital; Booming Trade in Forged Travel Documents Used by Criminal Underworld." Associated Press, 2005.

Taussig, Michael T. *Shamanism, Colonialism, and the Wild Man: A Study in Terror and Healing.* Chicago: University of Chicago Press, 1986.

The League of Nations in Retrospect: Proceedings of the Symposium. United Nations Library, Geneva Serial Publications, series E: Guides and Studies. Berlin: de Gruyter, 1983.

Thesiger, Wilfred. *The Marsh Arabs*, 2e. London: HarperCollins, 1985.

Tibawi, A. L. *American Interests in Syria 1800–1901*. Gloucestershire, England: Clarendon, 1966.

Tripp, Charles. *A History of Iraq*. Cambridge: Cambridge University Press, 2000.

Uhlmann, Chris. "Iraq Close to Ungovernable." *ABC*, March 11, 2014. http://www.abc.net.au/am/content/2014/s3960668.htm.

US Congress. "U.S. Committee for Refugees World Refugee Survey 1997—Saudi Arabia." Refworld, 1997. http://www.refworld.org/docid/3ae6a8ba14.html.

Van Heyningen, Elizabeth. *The Concentration Camps of the Anglo-Boer War: A Social History*. Johannesburg, South Africa: Jacana Media, 2013.

Vaughan, Megan. "Health and Hegemony: Representation of Disease and the Creation of the Colonial Subject in Nyasaland." *Contesting Colonial Hegemony: State and Society in Africa and India*, eds. Dagmar Engels and Shula Marks. London: Tauris, n.d.

Walsh, J. A., and K. S. Warren. "Selective Primary Health Care: An Interim Strategy for Disease Control in Developing Countries." *The New England Journal of Medicine* 301.8 (November 1, 1979): 967–974.

Webster, Charles. *The National Health Service: A Political History*. Oxford: Oxford University Press, 2002.

Weizman, Eyal. *The Least of All Possible Evils: Humanitarian Violence from Arendt to Gaza*. London: Verso, 2012.

Wendland, Claire L. *A Heart for the Work: Journeys through an African Medical School*. Chicago: University of Chicago Press, 2010.

Westrate, Bruce. *The Arab Bureau: British Policy in the Middle East, 1916–1920*. University Park, PA: Penn State University Press, 2003.

Whitehead, Clive. *Colonial Educators: The British Indian and Colonial Education Service, 1858–1983*. London and New York: Tauris, 2003.

Wilson, Arnold T. *Loyalties Mesopotamia 1914–1917: A Personal and Historical Record*. Oxford: Oxford University Press, 1930.

Woodyard, John. "Agenda: The Doctors' Malaise That Threatens Our Good Health/Shortage of NHS Doctors." *The Guardian*, 1986.

Zakarian, A. V. "Organization and Conduct of Mass Smallpox Vaccination in Iraq with the Aid of the Soviet Union." *Voprosy Virusologii* 6 (December 1961): 733–735.

Zaki, Saniha Amin. *Thikrayat Tabiba 'Iraqiyyah* [*Memoir of an Iraqi Woman Doctor*]. London: Dar Alhikma, 2005.

———. *Memoir of an Iraqi Woman Doctor*, ed. Ellen Jawdat. CreateSpace Independent Publishing Platform, 2015.

Index